THE TREATMENT TRAP

Rosemary Gibson
Janardan Prasad Singh

THE
TREATMENT
TRAP

*How the Overuse of Medical Care
Is Wrecking Your Health and
What You Can Do to Prevent It*

IVAN R. DEE   CHICAGO   2010

THE TREATMENT TRAP. Copyright © 2010 by Rosemary Gibson and Janardan Prasad Singh. All rights reserved, including the right to reproduce this book or portions thereof in any form. For information, address: Ivan R. Dee, Publisher, 1332 North Halsted Street, Chicago 60642, a member of the Rowman & Littlefield Publishing Group. Manufactured in the United States of America and printed on acid-free paper.

First paperback edition 2011

www.ivanrdee.com

The stories in this book are true and have been related to the authors by real people. In some instances, people's names have been changed at their request to protect their identity and their privacy. This book is not intended to provide medical advice.

Library of Congress Cataloging-in-Publication Data:

The hardback edition of this book was previously cataloged by the Library of Congress as follows:

Gibson, Rosemary, 1956–
  The treatment trap : how the overuse of medical care is wrecking your health and what you can do to prevent it / Rosemary Gibson and Janardan Prasad Singh.
      p. cm.
  Includes bibliographical references and index.
  ISBN 978-1-56663-842-5 (cloth : alk. paper)
  ISBN 978-1-56663-937-8 (pbk. : alk. paper)
  ISBN 978-1-56663-914-9 (electronic)
  1. Surgery, Unnecessary—United States. 2. Medical care—Utilization—United States. 3. Health care reform—United States. I. Singh, Janardan Prasad, 1960– II. Title.
  RD27.8.G53 2010
  362.10973—dc22   2009029352

To the one who makes everything possible

Contents

Acknowledgments

WE ARE ETERNALLY GRATEFUL to many people who helped us while we wrote this book. From the beginning, Peggy O'Kane shared her enthusiasm, which encouraged us beyond measure. We are enormously grateful to Helen Haskell and Deandra and Tom Vallier, who graciously shared their experience of medical overuse and helped us understand its impact. The book would not have been possible without them and all the other wonderful people we met who shared their stories. We honor them for their courage and fortitude.

Betsy Imholz, Chuck Bell, and Lisa McGiffert of Consumers Union had unerring faith in the importance and timeliness of this book. Their support and encouragement have been priceless. Friends and colleagues at the Dartmouth Summer Institute helped us understand the healthcare system from the inside and learn how profound knowledge, wisdom, and tenacity can solve seemingly intractable problems. We express our sincerest appreciation to Larry Jassie and Sarveshwari Singh, who read versions of the manuscript and shared their valuable insights.

Our publisher, Ivan Dee, saw the wisdom of this book and its salience in the current political context. We are grateful beyond words to him for making the book possible.

R. G.

J. P. S.

Foreword

AS I WRITE these comments, the summer of national health reform has become an autumn of complex political, financial, and emotional debates about the fundamental beliefs of Americans. Sadly, a major part of the discussion is driven by misinformation and the spreading of fears rather than a careful assessment of the challenges we face. We can only hope that efforts like Rosemary Gibson's and Janardan Prasad Singh's *The Treatment Trap* will enable Americans to view their health-care system differently.

From various corners of our culture we hear concerns that the assumptions we have made about health and our health-care system are incorrect. There is a growing sense that something else is influencing health care—not just for others but for every one of us. Gibson and Singh bring these valid concerns down to the individual consumer level as they tell the stories of Americans who trusted their health-care providers and the health-care delivery system only to find that they received care they did not need, at times with disastrous consequences.

Gibson and Singh share some experience that makes their approach to these issues especially relevant. Rosemary Gibson received a master's degree in public finance from the London School of Economics, worked as a senior research associate at the American Enterprise Institute, and then became vice president of the Economic and Social Research Institute. In 1993 she began her work at the Robert Wood Johnson Foundation as a senior program officer, shepherding several programs from launch to successful industry-wide implementation. She has earned special recognition for the leadership role she has played in the palliative-care movement.

Janardan Prasad Singh also has roots as an economist, focusing on policy work during stints at the American Enterprise Institute and the United Nations. He has advised many prime ministers of India and is now an economist at the World Bank. In 2003, Gibson and Singh wrote *Wall of Silence*, which examined the growing epidemic of medical mistakes. Their unique blend of economics, policy, and the real-world experiences of individuals makes them especially qualified to address the crisis of overtreatment.

For decades, Americans have believed that American medicine is the best in the world. The fact is that except for the most complex specialty health services, the United States lags behind many developed countries. On this larger scale we can see that the hundreds of billions of dollars in public, private, and personal funds we have invested have not led to medical success, financial stability, or individual satisfaction. We have paid an enormous price for modest incremental improvements and can now see that in many cases more medical care leads to worse health outcomes and financial destabilization for the individuals and families involved. *The Treatment Trap* brings to life this vexing problem in very human terms.

We meet Helen Haskell, an anthropologist, who lost her son Lewis to a combination of overtreatment and medical errors; her loss spurred her to crusade successfully for state legislation on patient safety. We meet Ron Spurgeon, a millwright and former firefighter, who found himself victimized by one of the most extensive overtreatment schemes in American health care. The authors interweave profiles with data and research findings that help us understand that the stories they tell are not exceptions but the all-too-common result of a dysfunctional system.

Gibson and Singh also introduce readers to a great many researchers, clinicians, and physician leaders who have devoted their careers to exposing the risky and wasteful practices of today's health systems. The current health-care debate has at long last included such experts, many of whom now find themselves in the thick of the reform process.

For the last several years, we at Consumers Union have gathered thousands of stories from consumers whose personal health-care experiences are compelling—and chilling. We have frequently found consumers whose problems in the health system began with overzealous testing or treatment. In some cases they have endured great physical and emotional suffering because of medical errors caused by procedures they didn't need. As in *The Treatment Trap*, their pursuit of the truth was stymied by a lack of candor, transparency, or caring assistance from a health-care system they should have been able to trust.

Gibson and Singh outline many useful approaches that individuals can take to detect and prevent overtreatment, and a range of systemic changes that could bring balance to a health-care system gone awry. At Consumers Union we share their call for constructive assertiveness when it comes to interventions that could be costly and risky. Americans should not accept errors, mistreatment, and excess as inherent to health care. We deserve better and should settle for nothing less.

Change will not be easy. In the 1990s consumers appropriately rejected a "managed care" approach to overtreatment that removed choice and created excessive financial incentives leading to undertreatment. In 1999 the Institute of Medicine issued "To Err Is Human," a landmark report that exposed the many unsafe processes leading to nearly 100,000 deaths a year. But ten years later there's been far too little progress, and discussions of safety in the health-care system remain largely behind closed doors. Few of the Institute of Medicine's recommendations have been implemented, especially those related to a more transparent sharing with the public of the frequency and effect of errors.

The Treatment Trap argues that we must begin to solve these problems by approaching health care proactively, not passively. We must understand the tendencies toward excessive or inappropriate treatment that too much money and misplaced financial incentives have encouraged. We must insist on transparency, explanation, and accountability—individually and institutionally. The Dartmouth Institute for Health Policy and Clinical Practice and the Foundation for Informed Medical Decision Making, for example, have repeatedly demonstrated that when patients are well informed they will make decisions that reduce overtreatment. Consumers Union's recent initiatives in rating drugs, health services, and hospitals have demonstrated that consumers want this information and will use it.

As I finished reading *The Treatment Trap*, I recalled Miguel de Cervantes' admonition, "He who loses wealth loses much; he who loses a friend loses more; but he that loses his courage loses all." This is a courageous book at a crucial time.

JIM GUEST
President and Chief Executive Officer,
Consumers Union, publisher of *Consumer Reports*

THE TREATMENT TRAP

Introduction

WE HOPE THIS BOOK will help prevent you from joining the ranks of millions of Americans who have become a victim of the treatment trap. Now, more than ever, you need to be alert to make sure you receive medical care that will benefit you. Here's why.

When we began to ask colleagues and friends a simple question—"Have you had medical care you thought was unnecessary, and if so, what happened?"—we never imagined where this question would lead us.

We heard stories that are quite common, such as duplicate tests, because health care is so inefficient. Other experiences were more serious. People described surgery and treatments that didn't make them better and actually made them worse. We read about a survey in which one-third of Americans say they have received treatments, tests, or medications they did not need. How could this happen?

We asked health-care insiders too, and they had stories to tell about their own personal experiences of overkill that had made them worse rather than better. They described how they had seen patients receive care that exposed them to great harm but offered little, if any, benefit. In fact, progressive leaders in health care who are deeply concerned about overuse say that many diagnostic tests, surgeries, and treatments are performed simply to make a buck.

In this book we introduce you to people who have had unnecessary treatment, and we share the stories of highly empowered individuals who avoided its pitfalls. Medical research that documents needless medical care is woven through the narratives, as is advice from health-care experts about how people can prevent overkill from happening to them.

In debates over health-care reform, a missing element has been the failure to confront the overuse of medical care. Politicians and the health-care establishment don't want to talk about it. One person's overuse is another person's payment for college tuition or a mortgage on a McMansion.

The stakes have never been higher for you to be smart about the health care you receive. Let this book be a guide along your journey to good health.

Americans are the ultimate consumers. The United States consumes more medical care than any other country in the world. Millions of people benefit—whether it is a heart healed, a fracture fixed, or a tumor treated. Healing is profound and unforgettable. The gratitude is heartfelt. Words cannot express the goodness of it all.

Then, why do so many Americans say they have had medical treatment they did not need? Is overtreatment real or are some people simply health-care nihilists who reject medicine?

Quietly buried in paper documents and in computer memory are findings from medical research that are applied too infrequently for everyone's benefit. Here are a few examples:

- One-third of people who were told they needed heart bypass surgery did not need it, according to research conducted by doctors at the Harvard School of Public Health and the Rand Corporation.

- People who have a full-body CT scan are exposed to radiation at a level comparable to doses received by some of the atomic-bomb survivors from Hiroshima and Nagasaki, according to findings from researchers at Columbia University in New York.

- Nearly 300,000 women have healthy ovaries removed unnecessarily each year during a hysterectomy. As these women age, many may die prematurely because of cardiovascular disease and osteoporosis-related conditions, according to a study published in the journal of the American College of Obstetricians and Gynecologists.

- Tens of thousands of children have unnecessary operations every year in the United States to surgically implant ear tubes as a guard against ear infections, according to research published in the journal *Pediatrics*.

- Tens of thousands of people have back surgery for chronic back pain when the evidence for surgical success is virtually nonexistent, according to researchers at the Dartmouth Medical School.

- More than ten thousand surgeries performed each year to prevent strokes have dubious benefit and may cause more harm than good, according to researchers at the Mount Sinai School of Medicine in New York.

- Ten million women have unnecessary Pap smears to screen for cervical cancer, yet they are not at risk for the disease because they have had a complete hysterectomy and no longer have a cervix, according to a study published in the *Journal of the American Medical Association*.

We asked doctors, nurses, and hospital CEOs about the unnecessary medical treatment they see from inside the health-care system. Their initial response was often a personal story, and they were eager to share their experiences as patients who had received medical care that didn't make them better and sometimes made them worse.

Some doctors have an unwavering confidence in the possibilities of medicine. Others are more skeptical and see the pitfalls. Patients too have their beliefs. Many Americans have a profound faith in the power of modern medicine while untold numbers of others are wary of modern health care and refrain from using the system when they can.

Nurses spend the most time with patients—more than physicians—and see the impact of medical treatment. As quiet witnesses to humanity at its most vulnerable moments, their minds and hearts are filled with memories of patients for whom the system did not know when to stop.

Health-care insiders confirm that medical care that doesn't make people better has become more prevalent in the past decade. The depth of concern is almost visceral. A seasoned nurse observes, "Health insurance used to be about giving people access to health care. Now it's about giving providers access to patients." The former CEO of Johns Hopkins Health System, Dr. James Block, says about overuse, "My God, there's so much. You see it everywhere."

Where is the fine line between appropriate care that makes people better and inappropriate treatment that does not? The line can be hard to discern because legitimate differences of opinion may exist about the scientific evidence for what works in medicine and what does not. Yet a consensus is emerging among progressive leaders in health care about medical procedures, tests, and treatments that are overused and do not benefit the people they are intended to help. In November 2008 the National Quality Forum, a Washington, D.C.–based nonprofit organization, released a list of prescription drugs, lab tests, diagnostic tests, and surgeries that are overused. The list includes antibiotics, x-rays, cardiac CT scans, heart bypass surgery, back surgery, knee and hip replacement, prostatectomy, angioplasty, and hysterectomy.

Most people don't become unglued about a needless x-ray or lab test. But seemingly little things account for a huge volume of unnecessary care and costs, and can trigger an avalanche of more tests and treatment. People *do* become unglued about major surgery that is ineffective or useless, and therefore unnecessary, because it invades the sanctity of the human body. It causes pain, sheds blood, and may trigger thoughts of one's mortality. The risk of infection and complications is ever present. Because unnecessary surgery provides a clear view into the world of medical overuse, first-person narratives from people who had surgery they never should have had are woven into the chapters that follow.

In part, this uniquely American phenomenon is a consequence of the overwhelming pressure to do more. Dr. Ethan Halm at the University of Texas Southwestern Medical Center has conducted research on medical overuse and describes the typical approach in American health care as "Don't just stand there, do something." In contrast, he says, skeptics of too much medical treatment say, "Don't just do something, stand there."

The "do something" culture is alive, well, and dominant. Americans live and work in a market-driven economy where businesses thrive on persuading you to consume more. The imperative is to sell anything—a house that's too big, a mortgage that's unaffordable, or a financial investment that sounds too good to be true. Market-driven health care is motivated by the same imperative, which is to sell tests, treatments, and procedures that are inappropriate, unaffordable, and promise more than they can deliver. Our bodies are scanned, prodded, medicated, and operated on more than any human bodies in the world. Our minds are marinated in media-filled medical hype and miraculous makeovers. We have been convinced that more is always better. The culture is fueled by a financial arrangement that pays hospitals and doctors more money when they do more. In the highly caffeinated health-care industry, the mantra is volume, volume, volume.

Dr. James Weinstein, director of the Institute for Health Policy and Clinical Practice at the Dartmouth Medical School, calls overuse an epidemic. As with any epidemic, this one isn't good for you. The pathogen that causes it is a mixture of money and human nature. One doctor calls it the "green monster." It lurks in every crevice in the system; its appetite is voracious, and it is obese. Policymakers in Washington who look out for the public's interest are trying to devise technical fixes to curb its eating habits, but it is infinitely cunning and constantly mutates. It wants to keep you in the dark—it doesn't want you to know that so much of medicine is guesswork. Under the guise of benevolence, it wants to sell just about anything to an unsuspecting public even if it doesn't help and may possibly harm. Its greatest enemy is the truth. It thrives on the fact that too little scientific evidence exists to justify a great deal of today's medical practice. In fact it wants to prevent good science from informing policymakers and the public about what really works because the green monster would be the biggest loser.

Overuse is the third rail of contemporary American health care. Politicians and medical leaders prefer to stay far away from it. That's because one person's overuse is another person's financial benefit. In this book we give voice to doctors, nurses, and hospital CEOs who witness it, and patients and family members who bear its consequences.

More medical care, not less, is an imperative for the sick who cannot afford it. It is an imperative for those who battle the faceless forces of insurance companies that deny legitimate claims. It is compelling for baby boomers who want to keep their hearts pumping, eyes seeing, joints moving, ears hearing, and brains remembering. All of us aspire to the blessings of good health. But this begs the question, "Is more always better?"

The Congressional Budget Office predicts that the United States could spend 25 percent of its gross domestic product on health care by the year 2025. Now we spend 16 percent. The federal government borrows money from China and other countries to pay today's bills. How will we pay tomorrow's bills if we can't pay today's? Unless the country changes direction, there won't be enough money to educate our children, protect our borders, or keep our food safe. Peter Orszag, now director of the Office of Management and Budget in the White House, testified before Congress when he was director of the Congressional Budget Office about the overuse, underuse, and misuse of health care. He understands this powder keg in the U.S. economy.

To take the guesswork out of medicine, unbiased research is needed to learn what works, what doesn't work, and for whom it works. You and your neighbor may have a similar medical condition, but a surgery or procedure may help your neighbor—not you. Your doctor may not know which of you would benefit. The American Recovery and Reinvestment Act of 2009, also known as the economic stimulus package, approved by Congress and signed by President Obama, included $1.1 billion to fund this kind of research. But public policy cannot and should not stop there.

Medicare and private insurers should stop paying for medical treatment that unbiased experts agree provides no benefit and may cause harm. The health-care industry and many in the medical profession prefer not to apply scientific evidence for the public's benefit because they would lose income. Whose interest should prevail?

Reform will require more than evidence and the removal of financial incentives to "do something." Technical fixes will be successful only if the political will exists to implement them. To create that political will, the impact of medical overuse on people needs to be seen and heard. That is the purpose of this book. It shines a light on the invisible people who are caught in the epidemic and are among the one-third of Americans for whom too much is done. We tell the stories that underlie the statistics. Here are a few examples:

A ninety-two-year-old New Jersey woman who was hospitalized and had a hysterectomy against the wishes of her family. She died a few days later.

A California man who had stents placed in the supposedly blocked arteries to his heart, and who was later informed by another cardiologist, "My God, you didn't need a stent. There's nothing wrong with you."

A woman who was given toxic chemotherapy for cancer she never had, one of several people treated by an Alabama doctor for nonexistent cancer.

In a spirit of optimism, we believe health-care policy can be made by the people, for the people. At its best, public policy is informed and shaped by human experience to remedy a social ill. The first step in reform is to give the human experience visibility and a voice.

Years ago the *British Medical Journal* published a commentary that said, in part, "From the ability to not let well enough alone . . . Good Lord, deliver us." May it be so.

PART I

Dare to Look

1 VOICES IN THE WILDERNESS

IT WAS 1998, and the truth was coming out. In Washington, D.C., the Institute of Medicine of the National Academy of Sciences convened a prestigious group of physicians, nurses, and consumers who acknowledged a uniquely American characteristic of our health-care system. They called the phenomenon "overuse" and said it occurs when the potential for harm of a health-care service exceeds the possible benefit.

What exactly is overuse? It happens when people have surgery even though their medical condition does not warrant it. It is the revolving door of seemingly benign yet unnecessary tests and office visits that can stir an avalanche of still more tests and procedures. It is the rendering of treatment when no evidence exists that it will yield a benefit.

The phenomenon began to be noticed in the 1970s when Dr. John Wennberg, a physician and pioneer in research on differences in health-care use among communities around the country, observed an epidemic of tonsillectomies in Vermont. His research showed that in the town of Stowe,

70 percent of the children had their tonsils removed by the time they were fifteen years old, compared with only 20 percent of children in Waterbury. Wennberg wrote, "For half a century, the tonsil has been the target of a large-scale, uncontrolled surgical experiment—tonsillectomy."

Wennberg discovered another epidemic, affecting men in Maine. Sixty percent of men who lived in certain communities had their prostates removed by the time they were age eighty, while only 20 percent of men had the surgery if they lived elsewhere in the state.

In the U.S. Congress in 1974 the House Committee on Interstate and Foreign Commerce held hearings on unnecessary surgery. Experts testified that nearly 18 percent of surgeries they studied might not have been necessary. In 1976 a House Subcommittee on Oversight and Investigations heard evidence and concluded that 2.4 million unnecessary surgeries were performed annually, resulting in 11,900 deaths. The annual cost of these surgeries was estimated at $3.9 billion. Since 1976, no new estimate of overuse has been calculated.

In the 1980s and 1990s the Rand Corporation and other researchers studied the overuse of selected medical procedures and found that many people had surgeries and tests they did not need. One of the procedures they examined was endoscopy, a most unpleasant examination in which the patient swallows a thin, flexible, lighted tube, called an endoscope, which then transmits a picture of the esophagus and stomach from the inside. Seventeen percent of endoscopies were performed for clearly inappropriate reasons.

The term "overuse" was first coined in 1991 by Dr. Mark Chassin, a physician and researcher, and now president of the Joint Commission, the Chicago-based organization that accredits and certifies sixteen thousand health-care organizations. In an article in the *Journal of the American Medical Association*, he defined it as providing a treatment when its risk of harm exceeds its potential benefit. At last a growing phenomenon in American health care had a name.

Although there was ample evidence of too much medicine, it did not arouse concern among the public, the medical establishment, or policymakers. "I feel as if I am a voice in the wilderness," says Dr. James Weinstein of Dartmouth, who has conducted extensive research on unnecessary back surgery. "There's a Latin phrase for it, 'Vox clamantis in deserto,' a voice shouting in the desert or wilderness."

OVERUSE COMES OUT OF THE CLOSET

In recent years, however, overuse has gained media attention. A *Wall Street Journal* front-page headline reported new studies that "hint at overuse" of stents to open clogged arteries. The *New York Times* reported on Elyria, Ohio, where the number of angioplasty procedures performed to open clogged arteries was four times the national average.

When Jane Brody, the veteran personal health columnist for the *Times,* described her painful experience with knee surgery, an orthopedic surgeon responded that his boss at his hospital complained that he didn't perform enough surgeries to bring in sufficient revenue. Brody wrote, "This is outrageous and just reveals the monetary motivation behind much of modern medicine. The patient be damned; just bring in the bucks."

Local newspapers provide a hometown flavor about overuse. In Hilton Head, South Carolina, the *Island Packet* reported on a whistle-blower lawsuit filed by a physician at Hilton Head Regional Medical Center accusing a physician colleague of performing hundreds of unnecessary heart catheterizations. The accused physician reportedly fled the country, possibly to Canada or Saudi Arabia.

The *Miami Herald* reported on a whistle-blower case brought by an anesthesiologist in which a neurosurgeon was prosecuted by the U.S. attorney for performing more than 150 unnecessary back surgeries. The *Minot* (North Dakota) *Daily News* described a lawsuit filed by a woman who accused a physician of performing an unnecessary lung surgery. That same month the *Victoria* (Texas) *Advocate* published an article, "Are Doctors' Morals for Sale?" quoting local doctors who claimed that their peers were performing excessive and needless tests and procedures "simply to make a buck." The newspaper alleged that "insured Victorians are being fleeced."

Consumer advocacy organizations have joined the voices in the wilderness to forge a path toward a more reasonable use of medical care. Debra Ness, president of the National Partnership for Women and Families, a Washington, D.C.–based nonprofit group that advocates for better health care, told a U.S. Senate committee, "Unnecessary care is rampant."

What lies beneath the news reports, congressional testimony, and health statistics? What happens to the people? A closer look reveals the untold human story.

2 A DOCTOR'S TALE

"GOOD MORNING TO YOU," the anesthesiologist said to the man wearing the goofy green gown that people are given when they are in the hospital. "Well, good morning to you," was the cheery reply from Mr. Goode, a grandfather in his seventies. The anesthesiologist who had been assigned to the operating room for Mr. Goode's surgery liked him instantly. "He was the nicest guy," the doctor recalls.

It was a Friday morning, and Mr. Goode was in the hospital for total knee-replacement surgery, a procedure performed more than half a million times each year in the United States. The orthopedic surgeon had told Mr. Goode that the surgery would relieve the arthritis pain in his knees, which made it hard for him to enjoy fishing, his favorite pastime.

As Mr. Goode was being prepped for surgery, a nurse came and said that the surgeon had just assigned a different anesthesiologist to the surgery. The anesthesiologist recalls, "I saw that my name had been blacked out on the schedule. The words 'Surgeon Request' were written on the schedule, which meant that the surgeon had requested a different anesthesiologist. I didn't mind the switch and spent the day with kids who needed their ear tubes replaced. It was a really good day."

By five o'clock in the afternoon, all the surgeries scheduled that day were completed. The anesthesiologist was on call and still in the hospital. A nurse called to report that Mr. Goode was coming back to the operating room. One of his legs was cold because it was not getting proper blood circulation. A vascular surgeon was scheduled to operate to try to restore blood flow.

The anesthesiologist remembers the next few hours. "I was preparing the operating room as Mr. Goode was being brought down. He looked a whole lot worse than early that morning. The big sunny smile was gone, though he was still very pleasant.

"I reviewed his chart thoroughly, which I would have done if he had remained my case that morning. His electrocardiogram, or EKG, suggested he might have significant coronary disease. In fact, if I had seen this EKG preoperatively that morning, I would have postponed the surgery to find out more about his condition. His medical record showed that no one had performed a cardiac workup.

"I asked Mr. Goode, 'Do you get dizzy spells? Have you had trouble with your eyesight?' He described an incident three months earlier when he had been driving and suddenly, but temporarily, lost his vision. He pulled the car over, and his wife drove the rest of the way home. I thought he might have critical blockages in the vessels supplying blood to the brain, a sign of carotid artery disease.

"I asked him about his legs and how bad the arthritis was in his knees. He said, 'The more I walk, the worse the pain becomes.' I thought to myself, arthritis doesn't get worse with more walking. Moreover, he was describing pain in his legs, not his knees. His condition was consistent with insufficient blood flow to the legs. In my medical opinion, he did not have arthritis. Peripheral vascular disease was probably causing the pain in his legs."

Peripheral vascular disease affects blood vessels outside the heart and brain and can narrow the vessels that carry blood to the legs, arms, stomach, and other parts of the body. Knee replacement surgery was not about to relieve the pain in Mr. Goode's legs. In fact, it appeared that his coronary artery disease, carotid artery disease, and peripheral vascular disease would make knee replacement surgery risky, and these risks had not been evaluated before surgery. This is why Mr. Goode was in trouble.

The anesthesiologist continued, "I question the medical judgment of a physician who would perform total knee replacement surgery on a patient with a medical history that had not been evaluated. I can't believe that the orthopedic surgeon did not know this patient was at risk. I believe I was taken off the case in the morning because the orthopedic surgeon knew that I would not have let the surgery go forward."

The anesthesiologist described what happened next. "As Mr. Goode was being wheeled into the operating room, I had a horrible sinking feeling. I tried to be upbeat and said to him, 'I'll be monitoring you and will give you drugs to help you relax.' I was very, very worried about him.

"While hooking him up to the monitoring equipment, I chatted with him and asked about his family. He said, 'You know, I love my family. I have a great wife and kids, but you never really understand love until you have a grandchild.' Mr. Goode won my heart. He was the kind of guy who would never have done a shoddy day's work in his life."

The vascular surgeon looked for a stretch of healthy blood vessel that he could graft and run down the leg to bypass the blockage in the existing vessels. Mr. Goode was under local anesthesia and could hear what the doctors in the operating room were saying. The anesthesiologist did not want him to hear about the difficulty they were having restoring blood flow to his leg. "I put him into a gentle sleep," the anesthesiologist said. After three hours the vascular surgeon concluded that he could not save the leg.

When the sedation wore off, Mr. Goode asked the anesthesiologist, "What happened?" The anesthesiologist replied, "You'll be going to recover in the coronary care unit, and the vascular surgeon who operated on you will come talk to you."

Mr. Goode knew the anesthesiologist was holding back. "I can tell something about you," he said. "You are a caring person, and you are worried about me." The anesthesiologist tried to dissuade him of any concern: "I worry about all my patients."

Mr. Goode persisted. "You are especially worried about me. I think I know why. I can tell you are really smart. I bet you are too smart to fall for that orthopedic surgeon's bull."

Mr. Goode's orthopedic surgeon had probably told him that the procedure was simple, that he would be home in a week, and that he would no longer have pain. Now he realized that the doctor should not have performed the operation. He was going to die, and he knew it.

Brimming with emotion, the anesthesiologist continued. "Mr. Goode raised his arm from the bed and tried to hug me. He said, 'I want to thank you for caring. I think I know what's going to happen. Do you know why I wanted to have my knees taken care of? I love to go fishing. And I couldn't go fishing because I couldn't walk. But now I won't be going fishing ever again, will I? I'll be walking in glory.'"

Later that weekend when the anesthesiologist was in the hospital, the overhead page alerted hospital staff that a patient had suffered a cardiac arrest. The code team was called to try to resuscitate him. The anesthesiologist recalled, "Mr. Goode came to mind, but I tried not to think about him. The following Monday I was in the operating room with a patient undergoing surgery and overheard one of the nurses say to another nurse, 'Did you hear about the total knee? He died of a massive heart attack.'"

"I had to sit down in the operating room while another anesthesiologist finished the case I had been working on. In all the years I have been practicing medicine, I have never had to stop in the middle of an operation. I tried to compose myself and went to the bathroom to splash cold water on my face. I have seen horrible things in my professional life, but this was the worst. The patient had risk factors that were never evaluated. A good and decent man had an operation that he never should have had. This wasn't a case of a missed diagnosis of heart disease. If Mr. Goode had had proper medical care, he would be alive."

The anesthesiologist confronted her physician colleagues. "As I walked into the anesthesiology department office, the chief of anesthesiology, my boss, was reading the newspaper. The anesthesiologist who let the case go forward was his cousin. I asked him, 'Did you hear what happened? The patient who had the knee replacement on Friday died. That surgery should have been canceled in the holding area.' The chief of anesthesiology said, 'No one important dies.'"

The anesthesiologist understood what he meant. People who are influential get good care. The little people, the seemingly unimportant people, do not get good care. Mr. Goode was a little guy, so he was not important in the eyes of these doctors. "They didn't see that once they stop caring about the little guy, the important people have to worry too," the anesthesiologist said. "If the system gets too sloppy, no one is safe, even the important people."

The anesthesiologist persisted. "I approached one of the orthopedic surgeons in the medical group who I thought was a decent guy and asked him, 'How could you let this happen?' He replied, 'Don't you see it? The green monster?'"

The anesthesiologist tried to fix what was wrong at this hospital but failed. The culture that allowed this unnecessary surgery to take place was too deeply rooted. "I put everything on the line to fix it. But I couldn't. Now I work in a place where we put our patients first. It's possible to put patients first and receive fair compensation for meaningful work."

Mr. Goode did not die because of complications of surgery or medical mistakes made during the operation. He died because he had surgery that would not have fixed his aching legs but instead exposed him to very great risk.

MANY DOCTORS, MANY TALES

When driving by a hospital with the familiar blue sign with a white letter H, the average person may see it as a place of benevolence. It is where expectant mothers rush when they are in labor, and where a high school football player heads if he breaks an arm during a championship game. A hospital in a community can bring a feeling of security; it is nearby just in case. Hospitals are indeed places of benevolence and hope. So much good happens within their walls.

Inside those same walls, doctors and nurses observe a different side of health care. Nearly 80 percent of doctors who serve in executive leadership roles in hospitals and medical groups and who responded to a 2005 survey conducted by the American College of Physician Executives (ACPE) said they were very concerned or moderately concerned about their physician colleagues overtreating patients to boost their income. When asked whether their colleagues were inappropriately admitting patients to a hospital to increase income, 54 percent of doctors who responded said they were very concerned or moderately concerned about this practice.

Although they are in leadership positions, physician executives seem powerless to stop their colleagues from providing treatment that yields no benefit and may cause harm. Autonomy is a cherished value of the medical profession. It gives license to doctors to do what they want, often without accountability. It is the driving force that compels high-placed executives to stand by and watch as their colleagues invite unsuspecting members of the public to leave the safety of their homes and be admitted to a place they would avoid if they could. This is autonomy run amuck.

The average person does not know what takes place behind the hospital's closed doors and whether he or she could be caught in the Bermuda Triangle–like maelstrom of American health care. Is the orthopedic department performing unnecessary surgery? Or is the cardiac unit doing unnecessary angioplasties, cardiac catheterizations, and heart bypass surgeries? As self-sealing systems, hospitals and other health-care settings have kept scrutiny of their practice at bay, whether it is oversight by their peers or by the public. No warning signs are posted to inform prospective patients they may be at risk. Doctors and nurses on the inside recognize the departments that do too much. From the outside, no one knows because no one is counting, no one is in charge, and no one is accountable.

Autonomy means that rules do not apply and are not enforced. In another survey conducted two years later by the ACPE, a doctor described the frequency of back surgery performed in his community: "Our community has the highest rate of instrumental lumbar spinal fusion, roughly 600% above the national average. . . . Expert guidelines are generally not observed. Inappropriate and unnecessary fusions are performed and far too many patients are left unimproved or worse."

Who are the people that did not improve and were made worse? What happened to them? Did those who had surgery know that they should not have had the procedure? How many more hospitals in the country have cultures like this, and how can the public know which ones they are? Answers to these questions do not now exist. But they should.

Mr. Goode was unaware that the hospital where he had knee surgery was a place with some good people who sought to practice medicine according to the highest ethical standards, acting with the benevolence every patient expects, and some other people who tolerated a different standard.

Patients win when good people drive out questionable practices; patients lose when questionable practices triumph. In the hospital where Mr. Goode had his surgery, ethical people lost the battle, though not for lack of trying. Their careers were threatened. They were labeled "troublemakers." The good doctors tried to hold the moral high ground, but in the end they lost the war. Mr. Goode was a casualty of that war.

The anesthesiologist who fought on the ethical side of this conflict and was so anguished about Mr. Goode's death reflects on medicine as a profession: "Medicine is the greatest. You can have a meaningful life. Helping people heal is the closest one can get to doing God's work. You relieve people who are in pain, and the gratitude from patients is extraordinarily rewarding. In medicine we have been given an incredible gift. But we are selling it for mud."

Mr. Goode believed in the power of modern medicine to help him live a good life as he grew older. By the time he grasped the ultimate betrayal perpetrated by the people in whose hands he had placed his life, it was too late. He did not see the "green monster" lying in wait for a seemingly unimportant and trusting person to cross its path and fall within its grip.

3 HOW DID WE COME TO THIS?

AMERICANS HAVE millions of surgeries every year. Whether it is a major or a minor procedure, each one is a memorable event in a person's life. The purpose may be to remove a skin cancer, repair a wound, replace an elbow joint, or recreate a face disfigured by injury. Tissues or organs are cut. A scalpel may be used, or lasers may beam a strong light to heat cells and cause them to burst. The National Center for Health Statistics reports that in 2006 more than 250,000 people had heart bypass surgery. Nearly 569,000 hysterectomies, 542,000 total knee replacements, and 231,000 hip replacements were performed in hospitals that year. Millions more operations are performed in physicians' offices and ambulatory surgery centers.

The widespread use of surgery today has been made possible by extraordinary milestones in its history. Among the earliest descriptions of cataract surgery, cesarean births, plastic surgery, and hundreds of other surgeries are those reported in ancient Sanskrit texts. The writings record the work of Sushruta, a physician who lived almost

150 years before Hippocrates in the sixth century B.C. He performed surgery and taught students the art of surgery along the banks of the Ganges River in the ancient city of Varanasi in northern India. Sushruta's writings and those of his students describe in vivid detail the techniques used to make incisions, extract foreign bodies, cauterize blood vessels, and amputate limbs. Methods of dressing wounds and using medications to prevent infection are documented. More than 120 surgical instruments and 300 surgical procedures are described. Suture materials were made from bark, hair, and silk; needles were made of bronze and bone.

When these Sanskrit writings were translated into English in the early twentieth century, the Western world had its first glimpse of the sophistication evident in ancient India. Sushruta is known especially for the surgery he mastered to reconstruct disfigured noses that used a flap of nearby skin, a technique similar to one used today by plastic surgeons.

MILESTONES

Thousands of miles away and centuries later in the United States in the mid-1800s, surgery was a dreadful last resort, an act of desperation. Mercifully, it was infrequently performed. The archives of Boston's Massachusetts General Hospital reveal that from 1821 to 1846, 333 surgeries were performed at the hospital, all without anesthesia. How unthinkable it is today to contemplate surgery without a shield from the pain.

In 1897 an elderly Boston physician reminisced about surgery before anesthesia, likening it to the Spanish Inquisition. The physician recalled "yells and screams, most horrible in my memory now, after an interval of so many years." In one of these operations, "the cancerous end of a young man's tongue was cut off by a sudden, swift stroke of the knife, and then a red-hot iron was placed on the wound to cauterize it. Driven frantic by the pain and the sizzle of searing flesh inside his mouth, the young man escaped his restraints in an explosive effort and had to be pursued until the cauterization was complete."

The first surgery at Massachusetts General using anesthesia was publicly demonstrated on October 16, 1846. The hospital's records note that the patient was Gilbert Abbott, a printer who had a tumor on his jaw. With an ether-soaked sponge and a glass inhaler, Dr. William T. Morton, a Boston dentist, administered the anesthetic, and the patient was rendered unconscious. A highly respected surgeon, Dr. John Collins Warren, removed the tumor. When the patient awakened, he informed the doctors assembled in the operating theater, in what is now the famed Ether Dome in the Bulfinch Building, that he had felt no pain. The *People's Journal* of London captured the significance of "this noble discovery of the power to still the sense of pain, and veil the eye and memory from all the horrors of an operation. . . . We have conquered pain."

After the achievement of surgery without pain, the next milestone was to reduce mortality from infections associated with surgical procedures. With little understanding of the importance of a sterile environment, as many as 80 percent of all patients who underwent surgery acquired infections, and about half of all surgical patients died from infection. At Bellevue Hospital in New York City in the mid-1800s, Dr. Stephen Smith was a surgeon and served as commissioner of health for the city. His accounts of surgical practice at Bellevue at the time are vivid. Surgeons rarely washed their hands before operating. During hernia operations, their unwashed fingers routinely explored abdominal cavities, and it was not uncommon for surgeons to invite bystanders to insert their unwashed hands into wounds for educational purposes.

Patients brought to the hospital for surgery were operated on without the surgical site being bathed, even if their limbs were begrimed with dirt. Surgical instruments were not cleaned, and when dropped on the floor they were simply retrieved and used again to amputate a limb or perform other procedures. Hospital floors were contaminated with a brew of human feces, urine, and blood.

Across the Atlantic around the same time, Dr. Joseph Lister, surgeon to Queen Victoria, observed that patients who had limbs amputated at home were more likely to survive than patients operated on in the hospital. Hospitals were far more dangerous places, he concluded. Lister was influenced by the work of Louis Pasteur, the French chemist and biologist who attributed the decay of flesh to microscopic organisms. Germs were the source of the infections the patients acquired in the hospital, Lister reasoned.

He pioneered antiseptic practices in surgery using carbolic acid, which dramatically reduced deaths from infection and heralded a new era of cleanliness and sterility. In April 1867 he reported that infections were entirely avoidable by antiseptic practices. Lister described a boy who had fractured his leg. Nine hours passed before he could be brought to the hospital, precious time during which multiplying germs could cause a great deal of mischief. Yet the surgeon reported that the boy developed no infections, and his bones were "soundly united" five weeks after his admission.

In the twentieth century, antibiotics, the sterilization of instruments, and microbial barriers were introduced to prevent infection. With pain during surgery eliminated and mortality from infection dramatically reduced, the stage was set for dramatic growth in the number of surgeries and their sophistication. Now, in the twenty-first century, surgeries are performed with robots named "daVinci" that remove cancerous prostates without a human hand touching the patient. Operations are performed on fetuses before birth to correct birth defects. Advances in surgery are a testament to the skill and commitment of physicians and researchers, and their relentless search to develop new ways to preserve life, add years to longevity, and improve the quality of those years. The patient's experience has improved dramatically. A Boston internist who was himself a patient says, "I had a complex surgery, and ten years ago I would have been in the hospital for ten days. Now, five hours after surgery, which was performed under general anesthesia, I was home eating ice cream."

With risks mitigated, pain eliminated, and virtually no financial constraints on the number of surgeries that can be performed, the United States finds itself in an unprecedented period in the history of medicine. Is it surprising that some of the millions of surgeries performed every year are unnecessary?

WHAT IS UNNECESSARY SURGERY?

Dr. Lucian Leape is a pediatric surgeon, now adjunct professor at the Harvard School of Public Health, who is nationally recognized for his work to improve the quality and safety of health care. He defines unnecessary surgery this way: "No operation is necessary if it is ineffective, if it does not accomplish its objective for a given clinical situation. . . . An operation is also unnecessary if it confers no clear advantage over a less risky alternative. In both instances the operation does not represent a net benefit to the patient. The patient will not be better off."

How often does unnecessary surgery occur? Dr. Leape reviewed published research that sought to measure it and concluded that about 10 percent of all surgery may be unnecessary. Where rigorous scientific evidence of the benefits and risks of procedures is unavailable, the percentage could be as high as 30 percent. Studies show that large numbers of operations are inappropriate and unnecessary. Here are a few examples.

HEART BYPASS SURGERY

As many as one-third of people who were told they needed heart bypass surgery did not need it, according to a study conducted by physicians at the Harvard School of Public Health and the Rand Corporation, where an expert panel of doctors provided a second opinion. During the study, reported in 2000, expert physicians reviewed a random sample of coronary angiograms performed at twenty-nine hospitals in New York State. Angiograms are x-rays taken during cardiac catheterizations to see whether the heart's blood vessels are blocked. A small tube is inserted into a blood vessel in the arm or groin and threaded to the area of the heart or to the arteries supplying blood to the heart. Liquid dye injected into the tube is visible on the x-ray.

When the experts reviewed the angiograms, they concluded that one-third of the people who were recommended for heart bypass surgery did not need it, or else the benefit was uncertain. In addition, 17 percent of people who had surgery based on the recommendations of cardiologists may not have needed it. With 250,000 people undergoing heart bypass surgery every year, if 17 percent of them do not need it, 42,500 individuals each year are exposed to a high-risk procedure that does not help them and may cause great harm.

BACK SURGERY

Millions of Americans suffer from chronic low back pain. The United States has the highest rate of back surgery in the world, even though back problems in this country are similar to those experienced in other countries. A type of back surgery called spinal fusion has been performed with much greater frequency in recent years. During the surgery, two or more vertebrae are welded together to prevent motion between them that can be painful. The spine is not actually fused during surgery; it takes three to eighteen months to develop afterward. The number of people on Medicare who have had this operation has increased dramatically—300 percent in a decade. Yet the operation is often performed on people with chronic back pain, even though there is no evidence that it is a better alternative to exercise and other interventions to help them cope with pain. But the lack of evidence has not stopped doctors from performing the procedure, which can take as long as twelve hours.

The increase in spinal fusion surgery occurred after the introduction of new surgical devices such as screws, wires, and cages that hold the spine stable until the fusion heals. When injured workers in Washington State who had an operation using these devices were monitored, 64 percent of them remained disabled after two years, and 22 percent needed another operation. Before they were widely used, the new devices were not rigorously studied to determine whether they would enable people to enjoy a better quality of life.

One physician has observed about his own community, "The costs for a fusion run as much as $50,000 to $60,000 or more, and without evidence that it offers any advantage over conservative care, it is unconscionable that inappropriate utilization is tolerated. Yet the surgeons who perform these operations are among the most powerful in the community because of the revenue they generate, and no one is able to take them on without fear of reprisal."

EAR TUBE SURGERY IN CHILDREN

Each year 500,000 or more surgeries are performed to insert tiny ear tubes in children's ears to thwart ear infections. It is the most common procedure performed on children that requires general anesthesia. But tens of thousands of these operations may be unnecessary. This is the outcome of research conducted at the University of Pittsburgh and the Mount Sinai Medical Center in New York.

For decades, surgery to place ear tubes in children's ears has been standard treatment. A small incision is made in the eardrum, and small metal, plastic, or Teflon cylinders or tubes are inserted. The tubes drain fluid in the ear, reducing the risk of new infection. It was believed that hearing loss from chronic ear infections (in contrast to acute ear infections that involve a short yet painful episode) could impair a child's speech and language development. While no evidence proved that children suffered from developmental delays or that their development benefited from surgery, it was nonetheless standard practice.

Dr. Jack Paradise and his colleagues at the University of Pittsburgh wanted to know whether children had improved speech, language, and intellectual development following this surgery. Beginning in 1991, they identified more than six thousand infants soon after birth and monitored them closely until they were age nine to eleven years. They found that children with persistent ear infections who had prompt surgery to implant ear tubes did not have better literacy, attention, academic achievement, or social skills. Ear tubes might help only some children with a rare combination of persistent infections and extreme hearing loss.

How many ear tube operations are unnecessary? Another study estimated overuse of this procedure. Researchers at the Mount Sinai Medical Center in New York reviewed the medical records of hundreds of children who had the surgery. They concluded that more than three-quarters of them did not have a severe enough condition—as defined by the American Academy of Pediatrics—to warrant the operation. If these conclusions are applied to the rest of the country, 375,000 children may be having surgery every year that is unnecessary.

REMOVING WOMEN'S OVARIES

Thousands of women may die prematurely because their healthy ovaries are removed unnecessarily during a hysterectomy, according to a study published in the journal of the American College of Obstetricians and Gynecologists. About half of the nearly 600,000 women annually who have a hysterectomy also have their ovaries removed. This has been standard medical practice for women in their mid-forties who have a hysterectomy, even if they have no ovarian cancer or family history of the disease.

In an accompanying editorial, Dr. David Olive describes the medical dogma surrounding the removal of women's ovaries during hysterectomies: "The predominant teaching is that . . . [the surgery] should be routinely performed over age fifty-five. . . . Most of us practice according to this dogma, and many utilize the cutoff of age forty-five . . . for when to strongly advise the procedure." Proponents of this practice assert that it eliminates the risk of ovarian cancer. The ovary is viewed as an organ for reproduction and hormone production, and when these functions cease, they believe, the ovary serves no purpose other than to generate mischief. Critics of the practice say that ovaries are hormonally active even after menopause, though not primarily for the production of estrogen. Moreover the psychological and emotional impact of castration is profound.

Today the "ovaries go" in about 300,000 women a year who have hysterectomies. Dr. William Parker, clinical professor at the University of California at Los Angeles School of Medicine, reviewed twenty years of published articles on the question of removing the ovaries. "We thought we would find that there was not much difference whether the ovaries were removed or conserved," he wrote. Instead he found that women who have their ovaries removed have a higher risk of dying from coronary heart disease and an increased risk of hip fracture. That's because even after menopause, ovaries dispense hormones that keep heart disease in check and bones strong. Meanwhile the study found no substantial reduction in the number of women who died from ovarian cancer. So the risks far outweigh any benefits.

Thousands of women may be dying prematurely, says Dr. Parker. He explains it this way. Let's assume there are two groups of 10,000 women each, between the ages of 50 and 54. One group would have their ovaries removed while the other would not. By the time they reach 80 years of age, 858 more women will have died in the group that had their ovaries removed compared to the women who didn't. Forty-seven fewer women will have died from ovarian cancer.

Among women who have had a hysterectomy, those who have also had healthy ovaries removed has more than doubled, from 25 percent to 55 percent, since 1965. This is a remarkable trend for a surgery that may cut life short.

Since the beginning of time, when healers have sought to treat and cure human ailments, decisions about proper care have been reached by gathering information about the patient and combining it with the doctor's experience and judgment. The doctor may consult with colleagues who treat similar patients, and may review the literature describing the experience of other doctors and their patients. Whether a procedure is appropriate or medically necessary has been based partly on the practice of a majority of physicians in a community. This approach to medical decision-making remains widespread today, even after billions of dollars have been spent on research to find answers to what works.

About twenty years ago it was estimated that evidence exists for only 10 to 20 percent of medical practice. Pioneering physicians such as Dr. David Eddy began to study how doctors make diagnoses and recommend treatment. He concluded that "It is not possible for anyone, even physicians, to accurately process in their heads all of the information needed for a complex medical decision."

Medical decisions are fraught with errors and are made with a wide range of uncertainty. This is why so many people receive medical treatment that does not benefit them and puts them in harm's way. It explains why some communities have high rates of heart bypass surgery or back surgery while other communities have much lower rates. People who live in Mason City, Iowa, or Bend, Oregon, for example, are more likely to have back surgery than those who live in San Francisco. "When different physicians are recommending different things to essentially the same patients, it is impossible to claim that they are all doing the right thing," says Dr. Eddy, who was the first physician to use the term "evidence-based" in referring to medical practice.

In the 1990s there emerged a surge of interest in a new concept in American health care: what doctors do for their patients should be based on evidence of its benefit. To non-physicians it might seem surprising that such a fundamental concept was introduced so late in the course of medical history.

What can the average person conclude from this brief history? That many medical decisions can be wrong. And when medical decisions are incorrect, patients receive treatments and undergo surgeries that do not benefit them and may expose them to possible harm.

Dr. James Reinertsen, a Harvard-trained physician and former health-system CEO, wrote that the practice of medicine "resembles the Tower of Babel more than scientifically grounded activity. . . . We are losing our clinical autonomy in part because the public has learned that one basis for it—the power of our scientific knowledge—is not being consistently applied for their benefit." He is right.

The situation is not entirely bleak. Human beings are on a continual quest to alleviate pain and postpone death. Enormous human ingenuity and energy are devoted to turning uncertainty into certainty, or at least more certainty, and the unknown void is filled by searching, researching, and searching again. The search may bear abundant fruit or reveal little more than folly. The search for a treatment for stomach ulcers illustrates the cycle of human endeavor to turn uncertainty into certainty, and to advance from medical practice based on belief and dogma to medical practice based on science.

FREEZING THE STOMACH: FROM UNCERTAINTY TO CERTAINTY

Stomach ulcers have plagued millions of people around the world for generations. Until recently, a cure was elusive. The high-stressed corporate titan working under constant pressure was an archetypal ulcer patient, and physicians believed that emotional stress and diet were responsible for this painful condition—until the real culprit was discovered.

In November 1963, the month that President John F. Kennedy was assassinated, *Time* magazine reported a promising treatment for peptic ulcers. Dr. Owen Wangensteen and colleagues at the University of Minnesota Medical School had experimented with freezing the stomachs of people who had peptic ulcers. Patients swallowed a tube with a balloon at the end. When the balloon was in the stomach, frigid alcohol was poured into the tube. A stomach frozen in this way would secrete much less hydrochloric acid for several months, it was believed, and protect the lining of the stomach and small intestines from becoming painfully inflamed. Proponents such as Dr. Wangensteen predicted that the treatment would be safe enough to be performed in doctors' offices.

Entrepreneurs saw an opportunity even before a rigorous study was performed to determine if stomach freezing was effective. According to *Time*, "Enterprising industry put the machines into production, and now nobody knows exactly how many of them are being used—and misused—in the U.S." The *New York Times* reported around the same time that five thousand gastric hypothermia machines had been purchased by doctors to perform the one-hour procedure in their offices or in hospitals. Many people had this procedure performed on them before doctors knew whether it was effective. Stomach freezing for the treatment of ulcers was eventually discredited. A rigorous study compared actual freezing with "sham" freezing, and the procedure was found to have no impact. Stomach freezing was laid to rest. In its place, medications to prevent the production of stomach acid became standard practice, hence the image of the antacid-popping pain sufferers, pining for relief.

In the 1980s and 1990s an Australian physician, Dr. Barry Marshall, and a compatriot pathologist, John Robin Warren, investigated their theory that stomach ulcers were caused by an infectious disease. Warren noticed that certain bacteria in the stomach were present in almost all patients with stomach ulcers. Dr. Marshall sought to discover whether these corkscrew-shaped organisms, called *Helicobacter pylori*, caused stomach ulcers. He deliberately infected himself with the bacteria and learned that his stomach ulcers could be healed when antibiotics were administered to kill the bacteria.

In recognition of their discovery, Marshall and Warren were awarded the 2005 Nobel Prize in medicine. The Nobel Committee noted that they "challenged prevailing dogmas" with "tenacity and a prepared mind." Marshall had been ridiculed for many years by the medical establishment, which believed the dogma that stomach ulcers were a chronic condition requiring a lifetime of treatment. A Boston internist recalls, "We laughed at Marshall." It is now firmly established that *Helicobacter pylori* causes most stomach ulcers.

Albert Einstein once said, "One thing I have learned in a long life: that all our science, measured against reality, is primitive and childlike—and yet it is the most precious thing we have." Indeed, when good science prevails, medical procedures that cause more harm than good are curtailed.

LEARNING WHAT WORKS IN A DOCTOR'S OFFICE

Conscientious and dedicated physicians like Dr. Paul Miles, vice president for quality improvement at the American Board of Pediatrics, use science in day-to-day medical practice to learn whether they are really helping their patients. Dr. Miles recalls a medical student who came to work in his practice in rural Idaho during the summer and asked him a question that changed his career: "Dr. Miles, how do you know what works?" "That question began to haunt me," Dr. Miles says. "I realized that I was betting children's lives on my decisions and recommendations, and for the most part I couldn't answer the question of whether what I did worked." That was more than twenty years ago.

Dr. Miles began to rigorously examine the care he was providing his patients. One of his first efforts was to reduce the number of children who were having a new surgical procedure that he and the physicians in his practice believed was being performed unnecessarily by surgeons in their community. A group of ear, nose, and throat (ENT) physicians had developed a new procedure—endoscopic sinus surgery—to treat chronic sinusitis. The ENT doctors convinced health insurers to pay them $12,000 for performing it. After that, the rural Idaho community had one of the highest rates of this procedure in the nation. Dr. Miles and his colleagues believed that the surgery was expensive, potentially dangerous, and of questionable efficacy. More than a hundred children in their small community had had this operation each year. Dr. Miles says, "The CT scans for some of the kids looked pretty normal, and our pediatric group was upset that they were having surgery."

He describes what happened next. "The five pediatricians in our practice looked at our referral pattern to the ENTs for this surgery, and at how we defined, diagnosed, and treated chronic sinusitis. What we found surprised us. The medical student who came to visit our practice for the summer worked on this project and found that in a three-month period we had diagnosed chronic sinusitis in 150 children. One physician in our practice had diagnosed it 96 times and referred the patients for surgery while another doctor had diagnosed it only twice and recommended surgery.

"With this huge difference, we asked ourselves how each of us defined chronic sinusitis and learned that we had six different definitions. We also asked how each of us examined the children, and it turns out that we examined them differently. To our surprise, we learned that we were part of the problem of the increased number of surgeries because we were inappropriately diagnosing children as having chronic sinusitis, which led parents to seek relief with the new surgical procedure.

"While we were indignant with the ENT physicians performing these operations for what we considered 'an acute remunerative procedure,' the finger of blame came back at us. We developed a practice guideline and were successful in reducing the number of children in our community who had the surgery."

With several physician colleagues, Dr. Miles developed a set of three questions for physicians: Why do you do what you do? How do you know what you do works? How can you improve what you do? "Since then," Dr. Miles says, "my career has been about how to help pediatricians answer these questions and improve the care they provide their patients."

SURGERY TO PREVENT STROKES

In 1988 researchers at the Rand Corporation found that a surgery to prevent strokes was being wildly overused—32 percent of the operations were being performed on people for whom the risks were greater than the benefits. Ten percent of the people who had this surgery either had a stroke that debilitated them or died within thirty days. The surgery involves removing fatty deposits from the carotid arteries, which supply blood to the head and neck, to prevent blockages that may cause a stroke, or "brain attack." It is called a carotid endarterectomy.

Did the Rand study and other research convince doctors to reduce overuse? A decade later, Dr. Ethan Halm and colleagues wanted to find out. They reviewed more than 9,500 medical records of older adults who had the operation. Almost 9 percent of the surgeries were found to be inappropriate, a significant decline from the 32 percent found in earlier research. This trend is good for patients, says Dr. Halm. "If you provide high quality clinical data from randomized controlled trials that better define the patients who benefit and those who do not, inappropriate use of procedures drops dramatically." But the bad news, he says, is that almost 9 percent of people who have the surgery should not have had it. If the results of the study were applied to everyone in the United States who has the surgery, he estimates that nearly 11,500 people have this operation inappropriately and some of them could die or have a stroke because of it. Dr. Halm advises that people must be carefully selected for this surgery because for some patients the potential for harm may exceed the possible benefit.

HOW TO STOP DOING WHAT DOESN'T WORK

For many years the American Cancer Society (ACS) recommended that heavy cigarette smokers have annual chest x-rays to detect a possible lurking cancer. In a dramatic turnaround, based on good science, the ACS later changed its recommendation. This is a story of how science was applied to stop tests and treatment that yielded no benefit and could cause more harm than good.

The tale begins in the 1950s. Researchers wondered whether chest x-rays could detect lung cancer at an earlier stage, an important question for a disease whose five-year survival is at best 20 percent but more often about 2 percent, according to the ACS. Over the next several decades researchers conducted many studies to determine whether screening for lung cancer would detect it sooner and thus reduce deaths. It can take time to build knowledge about tests and treatments that are effective and those that are not.

In the 1970s, randomized clinical trials were funded by the National Cancer Institute and pursued at the Mayo Clinic, Memorial Sloan-Kettering Cancer Center, and other distinguished institutions. The key finding was that chest x-rays did not detect lung cancer earlier in cigarette smokers. The mortality rate of people who were screened and those who were not was the same. The number of early-stage and late-stage cancers did not differ between the people who were screened and those who were not. Researchers concluded that chest x-rays did not benefit smokers and were unnecessary.

This research had another unanticipated effect. In the studies conducted at the Mayo Clinic and Memorial Sloan-Kettering, forty people who were screened and diagnosed with lung cancer had surgery that revealed they did *not* have cancer. One of the forty patients died of a heart attack after the surgery. Since the studies were carefully done at prestigious institutions, experts believed that if widespread screening took place at hospitals around the country where the quality of care might be lower, the number of people falsely diagnosed and exposed to unnecessary surgery would be higher.

Based on this research, in 1980 the American Cancer Society stopped recommending annual chest x-rays to detect lung cancer in heavy cigarette smokers who had no symptoms. Because cigarette smoking is responsible for the vast majority of lung cancers, the American Cancer Society instead recommended that people not smoke, a dramatic turnaround that has helped to prevent cancer.

The application of science for the public's benefit can be immensely satisfying. In this example, a diagnostic test was found to be ineffective in detecting a devastating disease, and with widespread use could cause more harm than good. This knowledge was applied, and money and human energy were redirected to effective interventions to prevent cancer.

A major reason for medical overuse is the lack of unbiased research on effective procedures, and the failure to use the findings. Dr. Reinertsen encourages legislators and the public to tell doctors, "You claim that your profession is based on science. We have given you power because of science's miracles. Now show us that you can use all the science you know for our benefit." A golden opportunity exists right now to do this.

THEIR MONEY OR YOUR LIFE?

President Obama's economic stimulus package included $1.1 billion for research to compare the risks and benefits of different treatments for a particular condition. Everyone agrees that more money spent on research is a good thing. But agreement stops there. The legislation establishes a Federal Coordinating Council for Comparative Effectiveness Research chaired by the secretary of health and human services. Its purpose is to recommend and coordinate research, but the federal government is precluded from using the research to curtail payment for treatments that are proven to be ineffective or cause more harm than good. If the public's interest were paramount, science would be used for the public's benefit: Medicare and private insurers would cease to pay for treatments that do not work.

The fiercest opponents of this proposition are the people who have the most money to lose if the truth about what works and what does not is applied to health-care policy. Beneficiaries of the truth are the people who lie down on a gurney and commit their bodies in the hope they will receive all the goodness that humanity can offer. Who should win?

4 THE HUMAN FACE OF "TOO MUCH"

STORIES BREATHE LIFE into the sterile term "overuse." They compel us to feel. Overuse often occurs because we have ceased to feel. Only by feeling once again will we be compelled to stop.

Medical overuse can grow out of a noble intention and a genuine desire to help someone who is suffering from physical pain. It can be the product of a deeply held belief that medical intervention is effective. This is how it happened to a physician and former CEO of a world-renowned teaching hospital who had back surgery at age twenty-four.

"I was in medical school at the time and had sciatica," he recalls, "a pain that travels down the large sciatic nerve from the lower back to the leg. My mentor, a well-known physician in New York City, recommended that I see a prominent orthopedic surgeon and a neurosurgeon. Both were chairs of their respective departments in prestigious teaching hospitals. There I was, a medical student, listening to two department chairmen saying they could do spinal fusion surgery which, back then, was a devastating procedure.

"When I decided to have the surgery, I believed it to be the best thing since sliced bread. In retrospect I was foolish. I should have been more thorough, but I grew up in a medical family and trusted doctors.

"After the surgery I had less pain, but the recovery took months. For years I was very limited in physical movement and couldn't ride a bike or play tennis. It has taken decades to gain moderate flexibility. Forty-three years later, I still have back pain and spasms because of the surgery.

"Why did they do it? They looked at my back, they didn't look at me. If they had looked at me, they would have seen that I had just gotten married and was under a great deal of stress. I should have had exercise and physical therapy. To them I was a nail, and they were the hammer."

The CEO says he has no doubt about the surgeons' good intentions. "They believed the surgery would help me." When asked why surgeons did not see the impact it would have on his life, he says, "There's a denial about it. They are selective and use only the information that reinforces their raison d'être. God gives humans the capacity to deny. It's hard to get through life without denial because it's too painful. In medicine we are constantly on a tightrope and forced to deal with situations that are life and death. Because it's so painful, we can't keep it all in front of us. We can let only so much data in."

This doctor's experience illustrates the power of belief that underlies a great deal of medical overuse. As a young medical student who had grown up in a medical family, he had a firm belief in the power of medical care to fix a painful ailment. He trusted that the actions of his doctors would benefit him. The doctors who examined and treated him had a similar belief.

His realization that the surgery did not help but made matters worse occurred over time. Its painful and unexpected consequences chipped away at his belief. As a young medical student, he discovered this by himself; the road to discovery can be lonely and fraught with uncertainty.

Scarcely any doctor will admit to a patient that he or she performed a surgery that should never have been done. And few doctors will tell a patient that another doctor's surgery was inappropriate and unnecessary.

Prominent physicians, however, are beginning to speak publicly about medical overuse they themselves have experienced. These public expressions give legitimacy to concerns about medical treatment that does more harm than good. They may spark an awakening among listeners and invite others to reflect on their own experiences and talk about them. Telling the truth about the unspoken is courageous, and courage is contagious.

Dr. Don Berwick, president and CEO of the Institute for Healthcare Improvement, is revered nationally and internationally for his work to help health-care professionals learn how to improve the care they provide to patients. In a speech to several thousand physicians, nurses, hospital CEOs, and other leaders in American health care, he shared the story of the unnecessary and excruciating surgery to repair his right knee, which he had injured while playing soccer as a medical student. His kneecap became dislocated, reset itself, and later became dislocated again. A surgeon operated on the knee. The recuperation was agonizing and the operation unsuccessful. The young medical student's kneecap became dislocated once again.

Looking back on his painful ordeal, Dr. Berwick reflects, "As it happens, I don't think I ever needed surgery on my knee in the first place. I certainly didn't need the extensive, painful, since-discredited procedure that this guy tried on me for his first time. The . . . problem I had was pretty minimal, and now I think that a brace and some exercises would have been enough.

"I think I fell into the very trap that . . . in health care, supply drives demand without regard to the quality of outcomes of care. . . . Do I believe for a minute that that kind surgeon secretly rubbed his hands together greedily and cackled, 'Hee, hee, hee—another knee I can make money on. . . .' Not on your life. I'd bet my life—actually, I did bet my life, didn't I—that that surgeon believed he was going to do me good. I am sure of that.

"But the fact remains: now I know that I had useless surgery for a nonsurgical problem. My surgeon and I didn't know that then. I have a screw in my knee for no good reason at all. My knee got screwed unnecessarily."

The prescription for good care—and the avoidance of unnecessary and inappropriate treatment—is the routine and systematic collection of objective information by doctors about their patients' outcomes. When this information is examined in an unbiased way, shared among doctors, and publicly reported to patients, doctors will know whether their work has benefited their patients. More important, a fund of knowledge will be built about what medical interventions are effective and what are not. And that knowledge can be applied for the benefit of many.

Socrates once said, "The unexamined life is not worth living." It may also be said that "Unexamined medical practice is not worth practicing." A thorough examination of the medical care provided to patients is one of the best prescriptions for health.

Your doctor tells you that you have cancer. Or your doctor says you have a ticking time bomb in your chest and at any moment could suffer a fatal heart attack. Imagine that you have surgery and find out later that you never had cancer or heart disease. A medical mistake, such as a mislabeled test result meant for another person, was not the cause. How can this happen?

RON, A CALIFORNIA MILLWRIGHT

Ron Spurgeon, a California native, served four years in the navy and was a firefighter for the California Department of Forestry. He has also worked as a boiler operator and a millwright for some of California's largest lumber companies. On Father's Day in 2001, Ron was helping his son with landscaping around the family swimming pool. While he was carting a wheelbarrow full of rocks, it flipped over. Ron could feel a twinge in his right shoulder but didn't think anything of it.

The next morning Ron woke as usual at 5 A.M. to go to work. He and his millwright crew were building an addition on a mill, and they had a nine-hour day ahead of them. As he picked up his work boots, he felt as if he had hit a nerve in his right elbow. The boots dropped from his right hand, and he could feel the pain radiate all the way up to his shoulder. Having had many perfect attendance awards, he was reluctant to miss work and break his streak. But his wife, Carole, called their family doctor to make an appointment.

The phone call set off a cascade of unforgettable events. Ron's doctor recommended that he see a cardiologist for a nuclear stress test to find out how well blood was flowing to his heart. He recalls the doctor saying, "This cardiologist is the best. He's a great man, and you are lucky to get an appointment with him on such short notice. If there is a problem, he will find it."

When Ron had finished the test, he asked the young man who conducted it, "Did I pass or fail?" He was told, "You've got the blood pressure of a teenager!" Ron went to the waiting room where he told his wife that the tests were not likely to find anything wrong.

Forty-five minutes later, the cardiologist said, "Sir, you have some serious problems. I think you've had a mild heart attack." Completely shocked, Ron asked, "When?" The doctor replied, "I can't tell. But you have a serious heart problem. We need to do a heart catheterization. You don't realize how bad you are. I should admit you."

A heart catheterization determines pressure and blood flow in the heart's chambers and reveals whether to treat blocked arteries with medications, a stent, or, as a last resort, coronary artery bypass surgery. The catheterization results showed that Ron's heart was in worse shape than the doctor thought. He needed heart surgery to bypass two or three arteries. He was admitted to the hospital immediately.

Ron recalls, "When my wife heard the news, she started crying. 'Is this how it's all going to end?' she asked. I said to her, 'I'm sorry, honey.' The look on her face and my two sons hurt me more than anything."

Reeling from the diagnosis, Ron asked his wife, "What do you think of all this?" She said, "It looks like you're going to have heart surgery." Ron still believed he hadn't had a heart attack. "It's pretty scary that you are on the verge of dying and don't know it," he says.

Ron was in surgery for more than five hours and had a triple bypass. The day after surgery, he recalls, "I was on enough medication that I didn't feel any real pain until the first time I coughed, and that's when I learned to love the pillow they gave me to hug."

During cardiac bypass surgery, doctors use a saw to cut open the sternum. The ribs are pulled back to allow access to the heart. After the arteries are bypassed, the sternum is wired back together again, and the chest is sewn shut. As many as 5 percent of people who have bypass surgery have complications, including death. As with any surgery, there are risks of infection and heavy bleeding. Patients may also have adverse reactions to the anesthesia and medications.

When Ron was ready to come home from the hospital, the surgeon came to see him and asked how he was feeling. Ron said he was looking forward to being at home on the Fourth of July with his family. He asked the doctor, "Can you tell me what was wrong with my heart and what the surgery did to fix it?" The doctor said Ron had been diagnosed with a "widow maker"—a severe stenosis, or narrowing, of the left main coronary artery, a critical artery that supplies blood to the heart. In surgery the artery was bypassed, removing the danger to his heart. His next heart attack would have killed him. Ron didn't know whether to start crying or hug this man for what he had done for him. He just said, "Thank you, Doctor." Ron recalls, "What else do you say to someone who just told you he saved your life?"

The same year that Ron had heart bypass surgery, doctors at Dartmouth Medical School analyzed information on heart bypass surgery rates in the community where Ron lives and more than three hundred other communities around the country. Ron had hit the jackpot: the rate of heart bypass surgery in his community was the highest of any in the United States that year.

Were people in his community older than people in other parts of the country? The data are adjusted to account for differences in age and gender, so this was not a factor. Perhaps Californians have more bypass surgeries than the rest of the country. They do not, and in fact the rate of bypass surgery in California is lower than the national average. If Ron's community were a medical destination for patients from around the country or the world, as is the Mayo Clinic in Rochester, Minnesota, or Johns Hopkins in Baltimore, this might explain the higher-than-average surgery rates, but it isn't a go-to place for bypass surgery.

Not only was the rate of bypass surgery in Ron's community off the charts, it had doubled from 1992 to 2001. Was there a sudden epidemic of clogged arteries? No, there wasn't. The hospital was performing surgeries on people who did not need them. Like a lighthouse in the fog, the information from Dartmouth was warning patients of rocky shoals ahead. Ron did not get the warning.

Ron's son was a detective with the Red Bluff, California, police department. About a year after his dad's bypass surgery, he called him to let him know that the FBI had raided the hospital where Ron had been a patient. It was suspected of performing unnecessary heart procedures.

Ron went to see a lawyer, who obtained all his medical records and hired doctors to review them. They concluded that he never needed bypass surgery. Not wanting to rely only on the word of the doctors the attorney had hired, Ron asked a local cardiologist to review his records. This physician confirmed the judgment: "Your surgery was unnecessary. I wouldn't have even done a heart catheterization on you. I'm very sorry for what you have been put through. These records verify what a lot of cardiologists in Northern California have thought about that hospital."

Ron was one of more than seven hundred people who filed civil suits against the hospital, Redding Medical Center, and its doctors for performing unnecessary cardiac procedures. The doctors contend they performed only operations that were medically necessary. In total the hospital and the doctors paid nearly $500 million in fines and penalties. But the federal prosecutor declined to criminally prosecute the doctors or the hospital.

"It's as if we were in the bottom of the ninth inning with the bases loaded, and the prosecutor refused to go to bat for the people mistreated by these doctors," Ron says with dismay. "The doctors and the people who ran the hospital just walked away. It is mind-boggling that more than $500 million has been paid out, but no one did anything wrong! These doctors threw out the hook and reeled people in, and nobody said anything or did anything to stop them. And sure, they must have killed people. If I walked up to someone on the street and punched him, I would go to jail."

After the FBI raid, the number of bypass surgeries at the hospital plummeted.

Doctors do not usually interfere in other doctors' business. If they move against the herd, the herd may drive them out. They may be perceived as troublemakers. Membership in the herd offers protection. So doctors retreat to a place of safety among the herd and become bystanders.

The bystander effect is a phenomenon studied by social scientists. Bystanders look to see if other people will intervene. If everyone else is standing by, they conclude that they do not need to act, or they assume that someone else will intervene. They may be afraid to act if their job and livelihood are threatened. A physician who is chief of obstetrics and gynecology at a large teaching hospital on the East Coast remarks, "There are three kinds of physicians—those who are in it for the money, those who do it for the right reasons, and those who are watching to see who wins."

At Redding Hospital in California, courageous doctors tried to stop the unwarranted and risky medical treatment. They failed, and the herd drove them out. The person who successfully pulled the emergency brake was a patient, a Catholic priest, who was told by the doctors at Redding that he needed heart surgery for what he later learned was nonexistent heart disease. After he contacted the FBI, the unnecessary surgeries stopped.

Although the public expects health-care professionals to abide by a higher standard and to do no harm, the profession does not regulate itself and curb its members who stray. In this case the FBI, not the medical profession, intervened. The reason for the FBI's intervention was the fraudulent use of money, not the harm to patients.

Overuse has become the norm in American health care, and its manifestation has become bolder. The overuse at Redding Hospital was especially brazen. Many examples of medical overuse are more subtle.

TOM, A LAWYER FROM OREGON

If any disease strikes fear in hearts and minds in the twenty-first century, it is cancer. The "C" word conjures up images too horrible to imagine, and worst of all, premonitions of one's demise. For these reasons the pronouncement of a diagnosis of cancer must be made with great care. To do otherwise is to inflict too great a cruelty. An incorrect diagnosis of cancer—because biopsy test results are assigned to the wrong patient—is an unforgivable mistake. The failure to perform a biopsy to confirm a diagnosis, and to pronounce a cancer diagnosis nonetheless, gives new meaning to physician autonomy.

Tom is a trademark and copyright lawyer from Oregon. He and his wife, Deandra, had lived in California where she worked as a production coordinator for a music company that recorded Chicago, Jefferson Starship, and Ozzy Osbourne, to name a few. Tom's clients included the Grateful Dead. Seeking more tranquility and green, open spaces, they moved to Hood River, Oregon, amid the stunning natural beauty of the Columbia River Gorge with its fir forests, blooming orchards, and wild bilberry. Their home overlooks the mountains surrounding the Columbia River, the land that Lewis and Clark explored.

Tom and Deandra undertook their own expedition in the health-care system. Tom had problems urinating and felt pain in his groin, so he made an appointment with a board-certified urologist. Tom had had a urinary catheter during a hospital stay the preceding year; the urologist told him that scar tissue might be causing his discomfort. He scheduled Tom for a cystoscopy. In this procedure, a small tube with a camera at the end is inserted into the urethra. A monitor then shows a picture of any stones, tumors, bleeding, or infection in the bladder. Snippers at the end of the tube can take a sample of the tissue for a biopsy.

During the cystoscopy the doctor called Tom's attention to the monitor. "Look at that, Tom. See that right there, that's cancer," putting his finger on the monitor on an apparent tumor in the bladder. "We need to get that out as soon as possible." He did not take a tissue sample for a biopsy that would confirm the diagnosis.

Tom was scheduled for surgery in three weeks. In the interim, the doctor encouraged him and his wife to come to his office so he could explain the surgery and answer any questions. "I want you to be totally comfortable with the procedure," he said. During the visit, the urologist drew a picture of the bladder and identified the location of the five-centimeter cancerous tissue. Tom and Deandra still have a copy of that picture. When Tom asked how far the cancer had progressed, the doctor said he would know only when he did the surgery and could see how deeply it was embedded in the bladder wall.

After meeting with the urologist, Deandra called the case manager who worked for their health insurer, a woman who was enormously helpful to them when Tom had been hospitalized earlier. Deandra recalls saying to her, "I can't believe it! Now Tom has bladder cancer!" A cancer survivor herself and a nurse, the case manager replied, "You don't know that. Let's get all the information before coming to a conclusion. You must have a pathology report. When all the cards are on the table, then we'll know what to do."

Deandra is a very savvy person, but she told the case manager, "He's the doctor, and he should know if it's cancer. How can a doctor ever lie about a diagnosis of cancer?"

Why would an intelligent, pro-active couple not insist on a biopsy? The case manager understands. "People use a lot of energy dealing with the threat of disease," she says. "You lose the ability to think clearly."

Deandra was worried sick that Tom would not make it through the surgery. The preceding year he had been hospitalized after falling off the roof of his house while cleaning the gutters. He hurt his back and broke his leg, and what should have been a one-week sojourn in the hospital became a two-month stay and a never-ending nightmare of mistakes and infections that almost killed him.

Now, faced with her husband's cancer diagnosis, Deandra was "hanging onto a cliff by a fingernail," says the case manager. "After a while your heart just breaks so much, and you don't have any energy left to challenge the information given to you." Deandra says, "After all that Tom had been through, I had no faith that he would come out alive. I thought he was going to have a heart attack and die on the table. I was sick for days, just beside myself."

Tom had a transurethral resection performed under general anesthesia at a local hospital. In early bladder cancer, the tumor can be removed using instruments inserted through the urethra. The operation was uneventful, and the surgeon announced, "It's good news. It was scar tissue. There's no cancer."

Instead of being overjoyed, Tom and Deandra were furious. They suspected that the urologist knew all along it was scar tissue and that the surgery was unnecessary. At Tom's follow-up appointment with the urologist, Deandra told him point-blank, "You shouldn't tell people they have cancer without doing a biopsy." The doctor replied, "Your husband saw what I saw on the monitor."

Deandra was too polite to tell him what she was really thinking—that her husband would not know the difference between a tumor and a hemorrhoid. "It was my belief, my medical judgment, that your husband had cancer," the doctor insisted. Deandra shot back, "Your medical judgment wasn't based on science. If you had told me that you base decisions on something other than science, we would have gotten a second opinion." The doctor replied, "I didn't mean to make you worry."

Deandra called the case manager at the insurance company and said, "I can't believe you would approve this surgery! Why would you pay these bills?"—which totaled more than $8,000. "We pay you a premium every month to look out for us."

The case manager understood the rules. "With your insurance," she said, "the doctor doesn't need preapproval for a surgical procedure if there isn't an overnight stay in the hospital." If Tom had stayed overnight, the insurance company would have required a positive pathology report.

"My husband and I felt so violated," Deandra says. "A doctor should never tell someone he has cancer if he hasn't verified the diagnosis."

The case manager took the unusual step of initiating an investigation. "We recently had an in-service training with our fraud investigation unit, and they wanted us to report anything that looked suspicious. In this case, I wanted the fraud unit to see if this doctor had a pattern of doing same-day procedures without a biopsy." The insurance company did not tell the patient or the case manager the outcome of its investigation.

Deandra wonders, "The doctor probably thought that everything would be all right in the end, and that by telling us it was just scar tissue, we would be so relieved. Meanwhile he makes money while we worry ourselves sick. How can a person be so spiritless, so evil? Some of these people are downright crooks! They have no idea the damage they inflict on people's lives. And this doctor is still out there."

MARY ANNE, A SCIENTIST FROM MASSACHUSETTS

Not all medical overuse occurs because of the opportunity for financial remuneration. Other forces motivate inappropriate medical treatment. Mary Anne is a scientist who has worked at the Massachusetts Institute of Technology and in the private sector. During her career, she had never thought that research in the pursuit of knowledge could be a stimulus for unwarranted surgery.

Uterine fibroids, or noncancerous tumors, develop in a woman's uterus. They can grow to the size of honeydew melons and weigh several pounds. About 30 to 40 percent of women over age thirty have them. Their cause is unknown.

When Mary Anne was told by her gynecologist that she had a uterine fibroid, she approached the diagnosis with the same energy and intelligence she devoted to her work. Her gynecologist advised that she needed a hysterectomy. Taking matters into her own hands, Mary Anne learned about alternatives, one of which is a myomectomy, a procedure that removes fibroids but leaves the uterus intact. This option might be for her, she thought.

The next step was to find a gynecologist who knew how to do the procedure to see if it would be appropriate for her. She scanned the Boston vicinity to find a physician who specialized in this surgery and found only a few. One seemed to be most promising. He was associate professor of obstetrics and gynecology at a major teaching hospital, taught at Harvard Medical School, published articles on fibroids in the medical literature, and was board certified in reproductive endocrinology. She made an appointment to see him.

During the office visit she remembers vividly how the accomplished physician had his feet up on his desk. One of his first questions was whether she wanted to be included in a study he was conducting to test a new drug treatment for fibroids. She declined and reiterated her request for a myomectomy. He recommended against it, saying that in her case the only alternative was a hysterectomy. Since he was the expert, she reluctantly agreed. With surgery inevitable, Mary Anne declared her desire to keep her ovaries, and the doctor agreed.

Because the operation was to take place at a teaching hospital, and fearing that a young physician-in-training might perform it rather than the seasoned doctor, she was emphatic that the senior physician perform the surgery himself. When she made this request, she recalls, the doctor stood up, banged his fist on the table, and insisted that he would perform the surgery himself. Mary Anne had complete confidence that she would be in competent hands. Finally, she wanted to be awake during the operation and asked for an epidural anesthetic. He agreed.

Nothing went as planned. Contrary to her wishes, Mary Anne was put under general anesthesia. When she awoke in the recovery room, she realized something was terribly wrong. Because of the pain, she was unable to lie flat. Her belly was distended, and she looked pregnant. A resident physician acknowledged to her that he had performed the surgery. When the time came to have her surgical staples removed, he did not know how to do it.

After she went home, she could not get an appointment with the gynecologist for more than two months. In the interim, another physician examined her but did not answer her questions about her excruciating pain. During that time she could not walk, stand, or lie down in one position for more than a few minutes because it was too painful. When she saw the gynecologist who performed the surgery, he did not examine her or answer any of her questions about her debilitating pain. He referred her to the sleep clinic that, in turn, referred her to a psychologist.

Once again Mary Anne had to take matters into her own hands. She found compassionate and competent physicians who discovered that dramatic muscle and nerve damage had occurred during the surgery. After a combination of physical therapy and medication, her pain has subsided but remains serious and debilitating.

Not long after the surgery, Mary Anne discovered that her doctor had been accused by the federal government's Office of Research Integrity in the U.S. Department of Health and Human Services of falsifying scientific data in federally funded medical research. The government concluded that the doctor had altered and fabricated information in permanent patient medical records and notes by changing dates, changing and adding text, and fabricating notes for clinical visits that did not occur. In one published study, 80 percent of the data had been falsified. The doctor confessed to these accusations and testified that he was pressured to conduct and publish research while also seeing patients two days a week, performing surgery one day a week, supervising residents, serving on hospital committees, and organizing national conferences.

Mary Anne also learned that the week before her surgery, the doctor made a presentation at a research conference in New York where he reportedly talked about the challenge of recruiting women willing to have hysterectomies as part of a control group for a drug study he was conducting for women with fibroids. She believes that when she declined his offer to take an experimental drug to treat fibroids, he recommended a hysterectomy so that he could nevertheless include her in the control group in his study.

The Massachusetts Board of Registration in Medicine suspended the doctor's medical license. The cause of this action was scientific misconduct, not the irreparable harm caused to a patient. Fourteen months later the suspension was stayed; he was placed on probation, and his medical license was eventually reactivated. He has resumed his career at a pharmaceutical company where he oversees clinical research in women's health. Public information about a physician's disciplinary record is maintained on the state medical board's website for only ten years.

Mary Anne's experience illustrates how scientific misconduct may have consequences far beyond breaching the ethics of scientific inquiry. Mary Anne has not been able to resume her career as a scientist because of the excruciating damage to her body caused by the surgery. The unwanted hysterectomy, conducted in the name of science without true informed choice, will have devastating consequences for her for the remainder of her life. She says she lives in a body that she sometimes wished "had gone to the morgue the day of my operation."

MICHAEL SKOLNIK, AGE TWENTY-FOUR

Not all people who have unnecessary medical treatment live to tell about it. At age twenty-four, Michael Skolnik of Colorado had what his parents believe was unwarranted brain surgery for a nonexistent cyst. From that day, Michael's life was never the same. The surgery was the beginning of a thirty-two-month nightmare of additional brain surgeries, infections, pulmonary emboli, respiratory arrest, partial blindness, paralysis, psychosis, severe seizure disorder, short-term memory loss, and multiple organ failure.

Michael became totally dependent. He could not eat, speak, or move anything except his right hand. During this horror, his mother, Patty, and her husband cared for their son day and night in their home. "Michael was unable to ambulate, was in diapers, had a feeding tube, was on oxygen. The list goes on and on," she recalls. "Injections each day, medicine mashed for the feeding-tube seven times in a twenty-four-hour period. Just turning Michael, who was six-foot-four, took three people."

His mother says, "Each day he pointed to his head and made a gun with his right hand to say to us, 'Shoot me.' He finally succumbed to pneumonia, and as he lay dying in his parents' arms he opened his eyes for the last time and mouthed the words, 'I love you.'" When Patty showed a video of Michael's nightmare to physician leaders in Colorado, they wept.

HOW OFTEN DOES IT HAPPEN?

Elizabeth McGlynn, director of the Center for Research on Quality in Health Care at the Rand Corporation, has studied overuse of medical care. "We have a body count for medical errors which grabs people's attention," she says, referring to estimates of as many as 98,000 people who die every year from medical errors. "We don't have a body count for overuse."

Dr. Lucian Leape at the Harvard School of Public Health has studied overuse and says, "Overuse is a serious problem. . . . We don't have a respectable overall number." Whatever the number may be, every data point is a person and a missed opportunity to do the right thing.

Ron, Tom, and Michael received potentially life-threatening diagnoses: "You have had a heart attack," "You have cancer," or "You need brain surgery." They and their families trusted; they believed they were being told the truth. Under such circumstances, it is difficult to question authority. Fear compromises the ability to think clearly and objectively. These individuals submitted to a higher authority because the figure in the white coat was the most important person in their lives at that moment, the one person who could make them normal again.

In the end, their experience was the exact opposite of everything they believed to be true about modern medicine. Their world was turned upside down. They trusted, and their trust was broken. For them, medical treatment was not benevolence, it was physical assault. By telling their stories, they can begin to make sense of their experiences, and others can learn from them. This is the human face of overuse.

WHEN WE SURRENDER

Dr. Richard Selzer, a retired surgeon and author from New Haven, Connecticut, provides rare insight into the unspoken voices of the patients who place their lives in the hands of the surgeon. In his book *Mortal Lessons*, he asks, "And what of that *other*, the patient, you who are brought to the operating room on a stretcher, having been washed and purged and dressed in a white gown? . . . In the very act of lying down, you have made a declaration of surrender. One lies down gladly for sleep or for love. But to give over one's body and will for surgery, to *lie down* for it, is a yielding of more than we can bear. Soon a man will stand over you, gowned and hooded. In time the man will take up a knife and crack open your flesh like a ripe melon. . . . Parts of you will be cut out. Blood will run free. Your blood. All the night before you have turned with the presentiment of death upon you. You have attended your funeral, wept with your mourners. . . ."

As we struggle to preserve our physical being, the need may sometimes arise to surrender it to the earthly gods for fixing and healing, until the final surrender to the earth. The body is the vessel of the spirit, so it is a temple of sorts. In the seventy or eighty years that it gives a human being a form with flesh and bones, it is a vessel within which one may find meaning, purpose, and joy in life.

"Doctor, into thy hands I commend my body" is an unspoken act of faith made thousands of times every day, in millions of surgeries every year. More than flesh is surrendered. Life itself is handed over, the life that is the form and shape embraced by husband and wife, mother and child. The surrender is an act of hoped-for love. Surely all human beings wish to know that when they surrender their bundle of cells and flesh and blood, they will be received with the same reverence with which they are rendered.

5 ARE YOU BEING NUKED?

THE MOST WIDESPREAD and costly over-use of medical care lies in the routine things—doctor's office visits, x-rays, lab tests, and referrals to other doctors. The churn of these items fuels a good financial return for health-care providers. While the office visits and tests may appear harmless, they can spark a parade of needless and unwanted medical treatment.

The domino effect, a concept from systems engineering, refers to a small change or event that triggers a similar change nearby, like a falling row of dominoes. The Vietnam War was viewed by its proponents as a way to stop the spread of communism in Southeast Asia. If one more country fell to communism, they feared, it would trigger a succession of other countries falling under Communist rule.

The domino effect also occurs in health care. Most people probably believe that an extra diagnostic test cannot hurt. In the 1970s it was recommended in the lay press that prospective joggers over the age of thirty-five visit their doctor to have an exercise stress test, to ensure they would not succumb to a fatal heart attack after they began jogging. Dr. Thomas Graboys of Harvard Medical School calculated the impact of this recommendation, and his findings were published as a letter to the editor in the *New England Journal of Medicine*. He estimated that if twenty million prospective joggers over the age of thirty-five had exercise stress tests, about 10 percent, or two million people, would have test results that showed narrowing of the coronary arteries. Exercise stress tests can produce false positive results—meaning the test can show that people have heart disease when they really do not—and launch a cascade of unnecessary tests and procedures.

Dr. Graboys estimated that the two million people with positive exercise stress tests would undergo cardiac catheterization, and about two thousand of them would die from known risks of the procedure, namely heart attack and stroke. Of the two million people, a fourth would have heart bypass surgery, and ten thousand of them, or 2 percent, would die from the surgery. In addition, forty thousand people would suffer heart attacks induced by the surgery. The cost of the tests and surgery was estimated at the time to be $13 billion. Dr. Graboys concluded that the recommendation for the diagnostic test could lead to personal and economic havoc.

The lesson from Dr. Graboys' calculation is that indiscriminate use of excellent diagnostic tools can have unintended and harmful consequences. When used properly, diagnostic tests can discover potential problems and save a person's life.

X-RAYS DESIGNATED A CARCINOGEN

Dr. Larry Jassie, a Bethesda, Maryland, internist, remembers the year 1980 when he returned to the United States after working overseas as a physician for the U.S. State Department for more than a decade. He cared for American embassy employees and their families stationed in Africa, Asia, South America, and Eastern Europe. Trained at New York University and Bellevue Hospital, Dr. Jassie is a physician who thrives on taking good care of sick people.

When he retired from the State Department, he began working as a primary-care physician in a group practice in Rockville, Maryland, and was astonished to see how American medicine had changed while he had been away. "I went to the clinic on a Saturday to review charts when a young doctor from the management team came in and sat down. He said, 'We've gone over your files, and you aren't ordering a lot of tests. Can you order more x-rays?' I told him that I take good care of my patients, communicate well with them, and have never been taken to court, so there doesn't seem to be any liability issue. I also said that if I missed something with any patients, we could review their files. He could not name any patients.

"I understood quickly the reason the young doctor came to talk to me. 'Compared to the other physicians here, you order a lot fewer tests than they do,' he continued. He wanted to increase business so the practice could make more money. I was stunned. How could medicine have turned into this? The doctor's office had become a business center. He wanted me to do more x-rays. It's basically criminal to expose people to radiation when they don't need it. If you didn't order enough tests, they would threaten to terminate you. I held my ground and continued to provide good care to patients, no more."

In 2005 the National Institutes of Health (NIH) included x-rays in its list of known carcinogens. Exposure to radiation from x-rays can cause breast, lung, and thyroid cancer and leukemia. The NIH report cautions that for patients who need x-rays and other diagnostic tests, the benefits far outweigh the risks.

Computed tomography (CT) scans are super-powered x-rays. From hundreds of x-ray beams, they create high-definition, three-dimensional images. The number of CT scans performed annually has skyrocketed from three million in 1980 to more than sixty million today. One-third of adults who have the tests are exposed to radiation unnecessarily, according to research published in the *New England Journal of Medicine*. Among children, more than one million have unnecessary scans every year.

NUKE YOURSELF

"Now taking appointments for February," said the ad on a popular radio station in Washington, D.C., shortly after New Year's Day not long ago. Capitalizing on fear, it asked listeners whether they wanted to know if a time bomb was ready to explode inside their body. Once the advertisement had listeners' attention, a solution was proposed. "We offer full-body scans" to provide peace of mind, a timely message since New Year resolutions are often health related. A full-body scan is painless and takes only about fifteen minutes. While a standard chest x-ray takes a single snapshot of one part of the body, a full-body CT scanner takes multiple snapshots as it rotates around the patient.

Surely every health-conscious person would have a full-body scan. Or would they? The advertisement did not mention a study conducted by David J. Brenner, a physicist and professor of radiation oncology and public health at Columbia University Medical Center in New York. He found that the radiation dose from a full-body CT scan is comparable to the doses received by some of the atomic-bomb survivors from Hiroshima and Nagasaki who had an increased risk of cancer.

Among 45-year-olds who have one full-body scan, one in 1,200 will die from a radiation-induced cancer later in life. According to Brenner's research, the odds of dying from cancer from a single full-body scan are greater than the odds of a person dying in a traffic accident. Annual scans for thirty years would catapult the risk to 1 in 50.

These risks are for patients who have no symptoms of disease. Organizations including the American Heart Association, the Health Physics Society, and the Food and Drug Administration say that the risks of a full-body scan for people who have no symptoms outweigh the benefits. But for people who have symptoms of possible disease and who are referred for medically appropriate reasons, full-body scans can be an enormously valuable diagnostic tool.

A research scientist who lives in the Northeast has a common heart problem, mitral valve prolapse, also called floppy valve syndrome. In the heart, the mitral valve separates the left atrium from the left ventricle. When the valve does not close correctly, a tiny amount of blood leaks backward, causing a heart murmur—an extra sound heard during the heartbeat.

Because the research scientist takes good care of her health, she went to a cardiology diagnostic testing center to have her condition monitored. An electrocardiogram measured the rate and regularity of her heartbeats, and a nuclear stress test enabled doctors to see her heart and how well it was pumping blood. It also showed whether

her arteries were narrowed or blocked because of coronary artery disease. The test is almost the same as an exercise stress test, except that patients are given a small amount of radioactive substance, hence the term "nuclear stress test." A camera takes pictures of the heart and picks up traces of the radioactive substance in the body. The pictures appear on a video screen.

"You are going to think I am making this up," says the research scientist, "but while I was having the test I overheard the cardiologist and a nurse talking in the test room. He said to the nurse, 'We're under pressure to get more patients. We're only at nine a day now, and we need to get to fourteen if we're going to make this place pay for itself.' I couldn't believe they were talking within earshot of a patient about the need for more business!"

She continues, "After the test, I was immediately a patient. The cardiologist was a brash young man in his mid-thirties. He said to me, 'Gee, that's a lot of PVCs [premature ventricular contractions]—do you feel them?' I told him that I know I have an extra heartbeat. He said I needed a mitral valve replacement, which requires open-heart surgery. He put me on a beta blocker and said I should stop running. Then he wanted me to schedule a cardiac catheterization right then and there. I knew I didn't want to have it done there, even if I needed it, so I left.

"I contacted a leading cardiologist, who had my electrocardiogram read by the head of an electrocardiography lab at a teaching hospital. He concluded that the test results were misread—I don't have a severe problem that requires surgery, and I don't need to stop running. I have a moderate problem that needs monitoring."

The fear induced by the doctor's diagnosis and treatment recommendations was palpable. "A diagnosis like this changes your view of your body and your life," the research scientist says. A planned family vacation was overshadowed by the dreadful thought of surgery, fear of mortality, and a radically changed self-perception—from being healthy to possibly facing death's door.

Who will be the five patients to make the diagnostic center financially viable? In the crosshairs of the medical arms race, the research scientist ducked a bullet.

Other unintended consequences occur from the feckless use of diagnostic tests. It is not an overstatement to say that overuse of diagnostic imaging tests affects everyone on the planet.

Dr. Fred Mettler is a physician who led the International Atomic Energy Agency team that visited Chernobyl after the nuclear power accident in 1986. He and his colleagues assessed the impact of radiation exposure on the health of the people living there. Closer to home, Mettler has studied the effects of medical diagnostic imaging procedures in the United States and concludes that they are the leading source of exposure to the American public of the most potentially hazardous form of radiation, ionizing radiation. In fact the American College of Radiology concludes that "the current annual collective dose estimate from medical exposure in the U.S. has been calculated as roughly equivalent to the total worldwide collective dose generated by the nuclear catastrophe at Chernobyl." This dramatic assessment demands immediate attention to the inappropriate use of diagnostic imaging tests.

To understand how a large volume of useless medical treatment is generated, an experienced and dedicated oncology nurse practitioner provides a rare look into a doctor's practice and what can happen behind closed doors. After working for twenty-five years at a large public teaching hospital, she wanted a change. She began working in an oncologist's private office practice, and here is what she found.

"When I worked in this office, the doctor made several changes in how he billed patients. Our patients who were on chemotherapy and taking the medication, coumadin, had to come into the office once or twice a week to have their blood tested. Coumadin helps prevent blood clots from forming in the blood, which can cause heart attacks and strokes. When patients take coumadin, their blood needs to be monitored because if bleeding occurs for any reason, it will take longer than usual for the blood to clot. The blood test results tell us whether the drug dosage needs to be adjusted.

"For the first six weeks when I worked in this office, I called patients on the phone to tell them their lab results and whether their coumadin dose should be altered. I would also remind them to come back again to have their blood checked. The blood test was the only cost to the patient.

"Suddenly the doctor decided that patients would have to come to the office to get their test results and be charged $75 for the visit. If they had health insurance, the co-payments would range from $15 to $30 or more. Patients had to drive, or have a family member or friend drive them to the doctor's office, and wait an hour or two to receive their test results. Some of our patients had to do this twice a week and travel up to 45 minutes each way. Just the cost of gas—it all adds up to a lot of money. These patients were sick, yet the doctor was really excited about this new way to make money.

"The doctor also wanted to increase his income by building a radiation practice. The patients knew they could get radiation treatment closer to home, but the doctor wanted to keep the business for himself. Our patients had to travel longer distances, and some had to travel the extra distance every day, five days a week, for four to eight weeks. I didn't have a concern that patients were getting radiation treatment they didn't need.

"The same thing happened with CT scans. Patients could get CT scans closer to their homes, but the doctor's practice bought its own CT machine to generate revenue and steered all the patients to it. When patients complained about traveling farther to the office for the scans, the doctor said it would be much better for them because he could view their scans online. In truth, we didn't have the ability to see the scans online. He would tell the medical assistant that we had to increase the volume of CT scans in order to increase revenue and pay for the machine. The medical assistant felt badly that our sick patients would have to travel so far. I noticed CT scans were ordered much more frequently than in the academic centers where I worked, which were prominent institutions. A case could be made that they were necessary, but they were in the grey zone."

This sort of office churn can produce more than increased cost to patients. The nurse practitioner recalls one of the most troubling circumstances: "A patient on chemotherapy was scheduled to come for another treatment. That morning the drug was prepared for him, but a blood test showed that his platelet count was too low to safely administer the chemotherapy. [Platelets are produced in bone marrow and help the blood clot and prevent spontaneous bleeding. Chemotherapy treatment wipes out cells in the bone marrow, and the platelet counts must be checked to make sure they have recovered before another treatment is administered. Chemotherapy should not be administered until the platelet count increases.]

"The patient was given the chemotherapy anyway and was placed at tremendous risk of bleeding. The drug had already been mixed and could not be returned unused to the manufacturer nor billed to the patient's insurance. Afterward the patient had to go to the hospital for a platelet transfusion, which takes at least six hours. I have never seen a patient's health compromised in such a way.

"I remember a gentleman we were treating for colon cancer. Every week, four days a week, he came for chemotherapy. It is exhausting, and patients have no energy to do anything else. This went on for months as the disease slowly progressed. We weren't helping him, but he was still coming. I believe the treatment should have been stopped, but with oncology, how can you prove that you are not slowing down the disease? At the very least, the doctor should have had a discussion with the man about stopping treatment and spending time with his grandchildren.

"Oncologists make most of their money giving chemotherapy to patients. The doctor would say to patients, 'I am not your doctor, I am your brother, and I'll be with you the whole way.' But the minute a patient decided to stop chemo and choose hospice, the doctor had no time to see him.

"It is a rare privilege to enter into people's lives at this critical moment. I love doing this work and want to do what is in patients' best interests. I left this practice after three months."

TOO MUCH OF A GOOD THING

Even the best of intentions can lead to overuse. About ten million women in the United States have had a total hysterectomy and no longer have a cervix, but they have had Pap tests and been screened unnecessarily for cervical cancer, according to research published in the *Journal of the American Medical Association*.

The Pap test is one of the most widely accepted and performed cancer screening tests. Routine screening for cervical cancer has led to a dramatic decline in cervical cancer rates and death. According to Drs. Brenda Sirovich and Gilbert Welch, authors of the *JAMA* study, women who have had a complete hysterectomy may not understand they are no longer at risk for cervical cancer. The National Cancer Institute says that women who have had a hysterectomy and have also had their cervix removed, and showed no cancerous or precancerous cells, do not need a Pap test. Yet the health-care system has become so good at screening for cervical cancer that it does not know how to stop when screening is no longer necessary.

Although the Pap test causes no harm, its unnecessary use wastes time and millions of dollars. Ilene Corina, president of Pulse New York, a patient safety advocacy organization based in Long Island, reviewed her doctor bill and saw that her insurance paid $36.41 for a Pap test. If this amount were paid for each of the ten million women who had unnecessary tests, the total cost would be more than $360 million.

PART II

Uncertainty,
Marketing,
and Money

6 UNCERTAINTY

THE IPHONE. A zero-emissions car. The space station. They have one thing in common: they are engineered with ingenious creativity. As their creators, humans know these objects inside and out. We are expert at fixing them. At our whim, we can take them apart and rebuild them piece by piece in any image or likeness.

After thousands of years, though, human beings are still trying to comprehend their own miraculous machine. Fixing it is not simple. Artificial hearts and joints mimic the real thing. Used parts such as kidneys and corneas are transplanted. Cameras are placed on thin tubes and threaded through orifices of the human body to see what is inside. Even as the edge of knowledge comes closer by the millimeter, it remains far in the distance. Belief, dogma, and enthusiasm about possibilities fill in the vast chasms of the unknown.

THE BASIC PROBLEM

"Uncertainty is a basic problem in medicine, day in and day out," says Dr. Paul Batalden, professor of pediatrics and community and family medicine at the Dartmouth Medical School. "Fear is associated with uncertainty. As a doctor, you are afraid because you have the responsibility for another person's life, and you don't want to cause harm."

Throughout human history, every generation has encountered uncertainty and come up against the boundaries of knowledge in preventing, treating, or curing diseases and conditions that afflict the human body. Each generation tries to break through the barriers and move from uncertainty to certainty, or at least to more certainty. In the process, rich and poor, kings and beggars, presidents in the White House and the man on Main Street are bearers of the consequences of uncertainty.

It was a cold and damp day on December 12, 1799, at Mount Vernon in Alexandria, Virginia. President George Washington had retired to private life after extraordinary public service that spanned military leadership of a revolution, the founding of a new nation, and the first presidency of the republic. As his public life waned, he returned to tend his farm at Mount Vernon.

According to historical accounts, it had snowed heavily that Thursday, and the wind was blowing. Washington surveyed parts of his eight-thousand-acre farmland on horseback from mid-morning until about three o'clock in the afternoon. Situated on a verdant bluff overlooking the Potomac River, the farm is out of sight and out of mind of the present-day seat of government twenty miles north in the city named for him.

Washington returned home that afternoon with snow clinging to his hair. The next day he complained of a severe sore throat. That night he had difficulty breathing. He asked his overseer, George Rawlins, to bleed him, a practice handed down from generations and believed to be a cure for a variety of ailments. Martha Washington urged that the bleeding cease out of an abundance of caution, but Washington allowed it to continue, saying, "More." His condition did not improve.

On Saturday, Washington was bled twice more. His attending physician, Dr. James Craik, sixty-nine and Edinburgh-trained, diagnosed Washington's illness as an infection of the throat. He was given a steaming mixture of vinegar and water to inhale. He was unable to gargle a mixture of vinegar and sage tea, nearly choking because he could not swallow.

A consulting doctor arrived, Dr. Elisha Cullen Dick, physician for the Alexandria, Virginia, board of health. A younger man, about half the age of Craik, he argued against another bleeding, saying it would weaken the former president. With still no improvement in Washington's condition, Craik bled him a final time, taking a quart of blood. The blood was reportedly thick and came slowly. Historical accounts suggest that, in total, at least eighty ounces of blood, or five pints, were drawn from Washington's body in about sixteen hours. The human body contains ten to twelve pints of blood.

Throughout the day Washington's health deteriorated rapidly. Drs. Craik and Dick wrote, "The powers of life seemed now manifestly yielding to the force of the disorder." Washington understood this to be true and said, "I feel myself going, I thank you for your attentions; but I pray you to take no more trouble about me, let me go off quietly; I cannot last long."

Unable to accept Washington's impending death, the doctors ignored his request and resumed their ministrations, applying a wheat-bran poultice to his throat. Nothing changed.

About ten o'clock Saturday night, Washington said, "I am just going! Have me decently buried; and do not let my body be put into the vault in less than three days after I am dead. 'Tis well." As he checked his own pulse, his hand slipped from his wrist. George Washington died on December 14, 1799, at the age of sixty-seven.

Modern accounts of Washington's death suggest that he may have died from acute epiglottitis, an infection that swelled the epiglottis, a piece of cartilage that covers the windpipe, and blocked his airway. Washington appears to have suffocated to death.

Today medical practice would require that Washington be admitted to the hospital for an emergency tracheotomy, where a cut is made on the neck to create an airway through an incision in the trachea, or windpipe. The open airway would have allowed Washington to breathe.

In Washington's time, bleeding was the treatment of choice for many diseases. The complications from the loss of a large amount of blood were not understood. "Today we know that many of their methods were wrong," wrote Dr. White McKenzie Wallenborn of the Department of Otolaryngology at University of Virginia's School of Medicine in his analysis of firsthand reports of Washington's final days.

In an uncanny coincidence, on the day of Washington's death a verdict was rendered in a courtroom in Pennsylvania in a two-year-old case involving the best-known physician in the United States at the time, Dr. Benjamin Rush, a signer of the Declaration of Independence. He had sued the editor of a Pennsylvania newspaper, William Cobbett, who had claimed that Rush, a proponent of bloodletting, had by this means committed medical malpractice and killed patients.

During the epidemic of yellow fever in Philadelphia that began in 1793, Rush had been an enthusiast for bloodletting and had proclaimed loudly and fervently the success of this treatment for yellow fever: "I saw no inconvenience from the loss of a pint and even twenty ounces of blood at a time. I drew from many persons seventy and eighty ounces in five days, and from a few a much larger quantity." Rush believed that the human body carried twenty-five pounds of blood. Cobbett described Rush's practice as being "one of those great discoveries that are made from time to time for the depopulation of the earth." Nonetheless, on December 14, Rush prevailed, at least in court. Cobbett was fined $5,000, a huge sum. But Rush was heavily criticized by his physician colleagues for his method of treating patients during the yellow fever epidemic, and was compelled to resign from the Philadelphia College of Physicians.

In a widely read newspaper, Cobbett wrote of the verdict, "On the 14th of December, on the same day, and in the very same hour, that a ruinous fine was imposed on me for endeavoring to put a stop to the practice of Rush, General Washington was expiring under the operation of that very practice."

President Washington's doctors had no evidence that bloodletting would be effective. At the time, medical decisions were not subject to systematic observation and analysis. A fundamental assumption prevailed that medical training, coupled with an association with similarly trained and informed colleagues, would yield the correct decision. This mysterious alchemy constituted the art of medicine. If the majority of physicians were doing it, it was the right thing to do. Even presidents yielded to their authority. Skeptics were derided and shunned.

In the throes of uncertainty, President Washington's doctors disagreed about the best course of action for the former president. Dr. Dick, the consulting physician, recommended a tracheotomy. Dr. Craik, the attending physician, disagreed. While tracheotomies are performed seemingly effortlessly on today's medical television dramas, in 1799 it would have been an experiment performed without anesthesia on one of the most famous men in the world. Craik assessed the risk in relation to the benefit and concluded that the risk was too great.

With the benefit of hindsight, Dr. Wallenborn wrote that if a tracheotomy had been performed, Washington might have survived the acute illness and lived for some time afterward. "However, this procedure was new and controversial, so they were not totally wrong to oppose it."

Uncertainty can fuel the imagination. Dr. William Thornton, a friend of Washington's and a physician, arrived at Mount Vernon the day after the president's death. He wrote in the 1820s of his idea to resurrect Washington's body, which had been kept in an unheated room and was frozen by the time he arrived:

"I proposed to attempt his restoration, in the following manner. First to thaw him in cold water, then to lay him in blankets, and by degrees and by friction to give him warmth, and to put into activity the minute blood vessels, at the same time to open a passage to the lungs and the trachaea, and to inflate them with air, to produce an artificial respiration, and to transfuse blood into him from a lamb. . . . I reasoned thus. He died by the loss of blood and the want of air. Restore these with the heat that had subsequently been deducted, and as the organization was in every respect perfect, there was no doubt in my mind that his restoration was possible. It was doubted by some whether if it were possible it would be right to attempt to recall to life one who had departed full of honor and renown; free from the frailties of age, in the full enjoyment of every faculty and prepared for eternity." In the end, the idea was quashed, and Washington was buried at Mount Vernon as he had instructed.

As humans seek to breach the boundaries of knowledge, a great deal of folly will be tried and tested. The brilliantly constructed mass of cells that comprises the human body trumps the deepest wisdom of the mortals. Until humans can fill the chasm of the great unknown, humility should be the guiding hand.

BELIEF

When uncertainty prevails, belief fills the chasms of the great unknown. Doctors and nurses who care for the sick have beliefs. Patients and family members too have beliefs. But these beliefs are rarely discussed.

Dr. Paul Batalden of Dartmouth reflects on his experience with two physicians who are both pediatric oncologists. "One believes that medicine does a lot of harm to people. He would fend off requests from families and discourage overuse, and he did this with the sickest of kids. The other physician believes in the possibilities of medicine, that it can do a lot of good, and that the possibilities should be explored. I would have my patients go to the first doctor because we share a basic concern about the hazards of medical interventions. Patients don't have a clue about their doctors' beliefs. Doctors often do not know the beliefs of their patients."

Faced with uncertainty, the doctors who cared for George Washington had different beliefs. Dr. Craik, the senior doctor and Washington's private physician, was more conservative; Dr. Dick was adventuresome and willing to try a tracheotomy even though it posed significant risk. Today, when patients and families hear a cacophony of conflicting recommendations from doctors, uncertainty and belief may underlie the discord.

Beliefs may evolve to become dogma, which is authoritative and reinforced by habit rather than science. For hundreds of years, bloodletting was dogma. Today, removing a woman's uterus and ovaries, for example, is often a matter of dogma rather than science.

Abraham Lincoln once said, "The dogmas of the quite past are inadequate . . . we must think anew and act anew. We must disenthrall ourselves." Lincoln's statement holds true for the practice of medicine. Medical care has an advantage over other areas of human endeavor with long-cherished beliefs: it can rely on science to disenthrall itself. But it must want to be disenthralled. Today, more than ever, beliefs and dogma are reinforced by financial remuneration, which makes the will to change immensely difficult.

ENTHUSIASM

Dr. Mark Chassin, president of the Joint Commission, claims that enthusiasm also contributes to overuse. When physicians and other providers of health care become passionate advocates for the services they provide, they are enthusiasts rather than objective caregivers whose recommendations are based on scientific evidence of what works. Enthusiasts truly believe they are doing good for their patients, according to Dr. Chassin, even though evidence exists to the contrary. Few physicians would knowingly expose their patients to treatments that could cause more harm than good. Misplaced zeal explains why overuse is not curtailed when evidence contradicts a doctor's beliefs.

This enthusiasm factor explains why Dr. Ethan Halm, in his study of inappropriate surgery to prevent strokes, found no difference in overuse between people with health insurance that pays doctors for each procedure they do, and those doctors in managed-care plans that have a financial incentive to curb inappropriate use. Dr. Halm also learned that patients who received care from the Veterans Health Administration had inappropriate surgery even though physicians who work in veterans' hospitals are paid a salary and have no financial incentive to provide unnecessary treatment. Financial incentives are not the only motivator of overuse.

FEAR

"Deeply imprinted in all of us is the fear of missing a diagnosis," says Dr. James Reinertsen. "This fear drives overuse." In teaching hospitals where future doctors are trained, young and impressionable trainees see patients whose community doctors did not correctly diagnose a disease or condition. "The spectacular failures of diagnosis become grand rounds presented by chief residents," says Reinertsen, "and there is a disdainful view of the doctors who practice in their offices in the community who miss them. You do not want to be the doctor who misses a diagnosis and whose case is the object of the chief resident's grand rounds." As a consequence, doctors who are uncertain order plenty of tests and bring in a bevy of consultants to help ensure that nothing is overlooked.

One kind of diagnostic error occurs when no disease is detected even though it is present. This is a false negative. The second kind of error occurs when a disease is diagnosed but is *not* present. This is a false positive. Most doctors believe that a false negative has far more serious consequences because an opportunity for treatment or cure is missed. Most patients also believe that false negatives are much worse, and lawsuits are filed more often because of missed diagnoses, not false positives. A New York cardiac surgeon, Dr. Irvin Krukenkamp says, "I order more blood gases, chest x-rays, and serum potassium than are really necessary out of fear that if something is missed it is a lawsuit." Doctors have less fear about false positives because of the perception that no harm is done, and whatever harm may occur from unnecessary treatment pales in comparison to the harm of missing a diagnosis and the opportunity to begin immediate treatment.

THE PEER FACTOR

Overuse can also be prompted by the expectations physicians have of one another. When primary-care physicians refer patients for specialty care, they may expect that the specialist will function as a technician and perform a particular diagnostic test or procedure. Rather than conduct a thorough and independent assessment, the specialist may be tempted to do as requested, even if it is not necessary. A physician at a teaching hospital explains it this way: "You don't want to offend the referring physician because you don't want to jeopardize future referrals."

COMPETENCE

A doctor's competence and diagnostic skill affect whether people receive the correct care, no more and no less. Dr. Eric Holmboe, senior vice president at the American Board of Internal Medicine, remembers a fifty-two-year-old woman admitted to the hospital for asthma three times in six months. She had been wheezing, a sign of asthma. Dr. Holmboe saw the patient for the first time during her third admission. He examined her and asked her questions about her health. "The patient's history showed no occupational exposures that would trigger asthma, she had no pets at home, and she was getting only minimal relief from the inhaler," he says. "They missed a heart murmur." He concluded that she had congestive heart failure.

At Cook County Hospital in Chicago, Dr. Brendan Reilly, a seasoned internist and geriatrician, reviewed the diagnoses and treatment recommendations made by doctors-in-training, or residents, for one hundred patients admitted to the hospital. Most patients had also been examined in the emergency department by an emergency medicine attending physician. Dr. Reilly conducted a thorough physical exam on the one hundred patients and studied how often the initial diagnosis and treatment had to be changed. He found that one of four people had been incorrectly diagnosed, resulting in unnecessary treatment for nonexistent conditions and delays in appropriate treatment. Here are three examples.

A patient who had been diagnosed with pneumonia and prescribed antibiotics was correctly diagnosed later as having the flu. The unnecessary antibiotics were stopped.

A patient diagnosed with an abnormal mass of cells on the neck had a surgical consultation. A diagnostic test was recommended. These interventions were unnecessary because the patient was correctly identified as having hypothyroidism, or an underactive thyroid. He was prescribed appropriate medication.

A patient had been diagnosed with congestive heart failure. A thorough physical exam discovered that the patient had a kidney condition, and a renal biopsy was ordered. The medication prescribed for the nonexistent heart condition was stopped.

Dr. Reilly is dismayed that young medical students and residents are not learning how to do a physical exam and do not understand why it is important. The human gathering of intelligence is needed, he says, for an accurate diagnosis, "preferably by a doctor who takes the time to look, listen, even touch. . . ."

What happens when good diagnostic skills are lacking? Says Dr. Reinertsen, "Doctors who are insecure and not confident in their abilities tend to order a lot of tests and hope something sticks." Patients bear the burden of incorrect diagnoses and the inappropriate use of hospitals, drugs, tests, procedures, and consultations with specialists for nonexistent diseases. Fear and weariness accompany each. The impact of it all is unseen, unknown, and unfelt—except by the patient.

KNOWLEDGE

People receive treatment based on what doctors in their community know how to do. If they do not know how to perform a certain procedure, patients may be overtreated.

In Richmond, Virginia, Dr. Thomas Smith, an oncologist at the Massey Cancer Center, inaugurated a rural cancer outreach program. According to Dr. Smith, the physicians in the rural area where he worked did not know how to perform lumpectomies, or breast-sparing surgery, on women with early-stage breast cancer. Instead women had mastectomies. Those who wished to preserve their breasts did not have the lumpectomy option.

In Dr. Smith's outreach program, the number of breast-sparing surgeries increased overnight when a respected surgeon, who was the director of surgical oncology at the Massey Cancer Center and also the president of the American Cancer Society, gave a presentation on breast-sparing procedures to surgeons in the rural community. He went into the operating room to help one of the local doctors do a lumpectomy. Afterward the percentage of women who had breast-sparing surgery increased from 20 to 70 percent.

EXCEPTIONAL COMPETENCE

Exceptional competence is an antidote to overuse. Dr. Selzer, the retired surgeon who taught at Yale Medical School, describes in his book *Mortal Lessons* an experience of exceptional competence. When a Tibetan monk, Yeshi Dhonden, the personal physician of the Dalai Lama, visited Yale–New Haven Hospital, he was invited to examine a patient in the presence of Yale physicians. The patient, a woman, had no visible signs of her disease. She was informed that she would be examined by a foreign doctor, and the visit was anticipated to be yet another in a stream of poking and prodding examinations.

Selzer writes of the manner of diagnosis by the Tibetan monk: "At last he takes her hand, raising it in both of his own. Now he bends over the bed in a kind of crouching stance. . . . His eyes are closed as he feels for her pulse. In a moment he has found the spot, and for the next half-hour he remains thus, suspended above the patient like some exotic golden bird, with folded wings, holding the pulse of the woman beneath his fingers, cradling her hand in his. . . ."

As rounds end, the suspicious onlookers and the Tibetan monk make their way to the conference room. He speaks of an imperfect heart and how, "Between the chambers of her heart, long, long before she was born, a wind had come and blown open a deep gate that must never be opened. Through it charge the full waters of her river, as the mountain stream cascades in the springtime, battering, knocking loose the land and flooding her breath."

When he had finished, the Yale physician pronounced his own diagnosis: congenital heart disease, interventricular septal defect, with resultant heart failure. The Tibetan monk's diagnosis was correct.

Is a human being's own acumen sharper than we know but lying fallow and weak from disuse? Dr. Selzer says, "Here then is the doctor listening to the sounds of the body to which the rest of us are deaf. . . . He is more than doctor. He is priest . . . the doctor to the gods is pure knowledge, pure healing. The doctor to man stumbles, must often wound."

7 MADISON AVENUE MARKETING VS. MEDICINE: A FAMILY'S STORY

AN EPIC BATTLE is being waged between medical science and marketing. Caught in the crossfire are innocent people, one of whom was a fifteen-year-old South Carolina teenager. The story begins from the moment an educated and engaged family read an article in their local newspaper, and ends with the realization that good old-fashioned science is no match for Madison Avenue marketing.

Like many families faced with a decision about surgery, Helen Haskell and her family from Columbia, South Carolina, tried to do their homework. They learned about an elective surgery for their son, Lewis, and asked the right questions about the hospital, the procedure, and the surgeon who was going to perform it.

Helen is an anthropologist, and her training prepared her to plan carefully. In Africa near the Niger River, she directed excavations of prehistoric communities in what is now Mali. Closer to home, she did excavations along the swampy South Carolina coast where rice plantations flourished in the eighteenth century from the labor of slaves.

Her son, Lewis, was born with "funnel chest," or pectus excavatum. The breast bone, or sternum, is pushed back toward the spine, leaving a visible depression, or funnel, in the chest. The heart and lungs of children with severe pectus excavatum may have a diminished capacity because of compression from the sternum, which can cause difficulty breathing when the child is physically active. But like most people with pectus excavatum, Lewis's condition was not severe and did not affect his health. Lewis was a top student in high school, a budding writer who wrote for his local newspaper, and an actor in community theater. At the age of seven he appeared in a television commercial with Dale Earnhardt, the late NASCAR driver.

"We first learned of a new surgical procedure for funnel chest in June 1999 from our local newspaper," Helen said, referring to the Columbia *State*. The procedure was described as a revolutionary and less invasive alternative to another type of surgery that opens up the entire chest. "My husband and I got the impression that any responsible parents would do this for their child," she says.

During the operation a metal bar is inserted through three small incisions in the chest. The bar is fixed to the ribs and props up the breastbone. After two or more years when the breastbone has remolded and straightened, the bar is removed. Helen had the impression that it was like getting braces to straighten teeth.

That summer, when Lewis went for his camp checkup, his parents asked their pediatrician about the surgery. According to Helen, the doctor told her he would look into it. A few weeks later he called and said he had had a long conversation with a pediatric surgeon at the hospital named in the newspaper article. He seemed to be impressed with what he had heard, and suggested that the surgery would be a neat little operation and good for Lewis. He gave Helen the name of a pediatric surgeon and recommended that she talk with him.

The family met with the pediatric surgeon in October 1999 to learn about the procedure. He was a big, hearty guy, and they liked him immediately. It was evident he loved children. His years of surgical experience instilled confidence in them.

When they asked about the operation portrayed in the newspaper, to their surprise he seemed to steer them toward the more traditional procedure that opened the chest. Lewis's parents were bewildered. They had come to the hospital because they had read about the less invasive operation being performed there. Helen said, "The hospital's website gave us the impression that the older procedure was draconian and dangerous, and that we should avoid it." So they never considered it.

During the meeting, the doctor said his department was doing a study of the new surgery at hospitals around the country. Helen asked for information about Lewis's condition and the procedure, and the surgeon gave her a copy of a chapter from a pediatric textbook that described funnel chest. He also gave her an article published a year earlier by a pediatric surgeon at a hospital out of state. The article concluded that the less invasive surgery was effective. Of the forty-two children who had had the operation, twelve had complications, all of which were reportedly managed with relative ease. The principal author of the article had developed this new, less invasive surgery, and was an owner of the patent for the steel bar used to prop up the breastbone. Since the procedure was relatively new, Helen assumed that this was the only article yet published.

A few days after the meeting, Helen wanted to know how many times the pediatric surgeon to whom she and her family had spoken had performed the new operation. When she called the nurse in his office, Helen recalls her laughing and saying, "Don't worry, he's done it plenty."

This reply stuck in Helen's mind because it seemed evasive. "How many is plenty?" Helen asked. "Oh, I don't know," Helen recalls the nurse saying. "About twenty. You really don't need to worry. He's done it plenty."

Helen and her family looked at websites about the procedure that described it as new, minimally invasive, and safe. They contacted two families referred by the pediatric surgeon's office and two other families they found independently, and all said the surgeries had been successful. Helen and her family debated the merits of the surgery for months. They did not consider that surgery performed on a child might be dangerous. In the end, they decided to go ahead with it.

The surgery was performed on a Thursday and took longer than Lewis's parents expected, but the surgeon assured them it had gone well. After the operation, Lewis was given a narcotic pain medication through an epidural catheter in his back. He was also given regular injections of a powerful painkiller, Ketorolac, which the family later learned was labeled with warnings in bold print about the possibility of perforated ulcers, bleeding, and kidney failure.

Early Sunday morning Lewis was stricken with the "worst pain imaginable," he told his mom. The pain was around his stomach, not in his chest where the surgery had been performed. Helen recalls that the nurses and residents told her and Lewis that the narcotic pain medication was causing constipation. As the day wore on, his condition worsened and his belly became bloated, his heart rate increased, his temperature dropped, and he became pale and weak and dripped with sweat. Helen repeatedly asked for a senior doctor to examine him. Because it was a Sunday, no senior doctor came to the hospital to check on Lewis. The young residents and nurses who took care of him continued to insist that he was suffering from constipation.

By late Sunday night Lewis's temperature had dropped to 95 degrees and his heart rate had soared to 142 beats per minute. Helen wrote in her journal, "Neither Lewis nor I sleep at all Sunday night."

On Monday Lewis's condition continued to deteriorate. Helen and Lewis waited in vain for the senior doctor. Helen later learned that he had never been called. Around noon, Lewis told his mom that the world was going black. In her journal, Helen wrote the last thing he ever said—"Ish . . . going . . . black." He repeated it again and passed out. "Suddenly, Lewis is dead. It is 12:05 P.M."

Ninety-six hours after he had been admitted to the hospital, Lewis died of a perforated duodenal ulcer. The autopsy found nearly three quarts of blood and other fluids in his abdomen. An adult weighing about 150 pounds has about four to five quarts of blood.

The pediatric surgeon, Helen recalls, acknowledged that a tragic mistake had been made. Lewis's death was a case of failure to rescue, a term used in hospitals to describe patients who die when clinical signs of their deterioration, such as elevated heart rate or loss of consciousness, are present but are not treated in a timely manner.

More than a year and a half after Lewis died, the *State* published a front-page story describing the events surrounding his death and pointing a finger at the lack of supervision in teaching hospitals. It was the same newspaper where Lewis's parents had read about the new, minimally invasive surgery.

THE FINE PRINT

Helen buried her grief in research to find out what had gone wrong with a surgery that was supposed to be so safe. She discovered Medline, an internet-accessible treasure trove of articles and summaries of articles sponsored by the National Library of Medicine, which is part of the National Institutes of Health. Helen says, "When I researched the surgery Lewis had, I was deeply disturbed at what I found."

The article the surgeon had given her was not the only published article, as she had thought, but was one of several reports on the procedure. Some of them revealed serious implications of surgery. "I could not believe we had submitted our child to the risks reported in the medical literature," Helen says.

Among the articles was a study whose authors included the surgeons from the hospital where Lewis had his operation, including his own surgeon. This was the study he had mentioned in their initial meeting. Helen was surprised to discover that it had been completed and published nine months before Lewis's surgery. It examined the outcomes of the new procedure among 251 children at 32 hospitals. The incidence of complications and problems was found to be "quite high (21%)." Side effects were reported from the powerful drugs needed to control the unusual level of pain associated with the surgery. During Lewis's hospitalization, drug side effects were not properly managed, leading to a downward spiral culminating in his death.

Helen found another article in which doctors at a children's hospital in Indianapolis reported that one-third of the children who had had the surgery needed a second operation. The authors concluded, "Despite the ease of the procedure and its simplistic nature, there is considerable morbidity associated with this learning curve that cannot be underestimated. Although previous reports suggest few complications occur, we believe that further assessment[s] . . . are still needed." This article too was published nine months before Lewis had his surgery.

Helen kept searching and found yet another study, published two months after Lewis's operation. Pediatric surgeons from Stanford University Children's Hospital, the University of California at San Francisco, and Children's Memorial Hospital in Chicago reported on five children who had suffered severe complications from the surgery, including an eight-year old boy whose heart had been perforated during the procedure.

Another article published three months after Lewis's operation found that nearly half the children who had had the surgery suffered complications. The authors concluded that the procedure had high complication and reoperation rates. Twenty-nine percent of the children needed a second operation.

Helen felt betrayed. She and her family had not been told about the extent of the risks of the surgery. "All my assumptions about Lewis's surgery had been based on a fundamental notion of trust," she says. "When it comes to surgery and other medical treatment, at some point you have to believe that people are telling you the whole story." When asked what she would have done differently if she had been informed of the risks, she says, "We would have done everything differently. We would never have taken our child for this surgery if we had understood the extent and severity of the complications."

When asked why she did not look for more research on the procedure before making a decision, Helen says, "I am a researcher, but I didn't know how to search the medical literature." The article the pediatric surgeon gave her said that the operation was effective and had excellent long-term results. Helen continues, "The irony is that Lewis's surgeon probably considered us to be among his best-informed families. We had pieces of information about certain complications, but it was not put together in a way that made the risks clear to us. We came away thinking that this was a safe procedure, that it had some relatively rare problems when it was first introduced, but that those problems had been corrected. The enthusiastic reports we had read on the internet and the hospital website all emphasized safety as a benefit of the procedure. This created a mind-set that made it very difficult for us to understand that it might not be very safe. In retrospect we were naive. At the time we didn't think we were. We thought we were well informed."

THE TRUTH NOT FIT TO PRINT

Eighteen months after Lewis died, an article in the *Journal of Pediatric Surgery* compared the complication rates of the less invasive surgery performed at the hospital where Lewis had the operation, and the traditional procedure, performed at a California hospital. The study had a striking omission. "There were no deaths" from the innovative surgery, it reported. The study included children who had had the surgery from January 1996 through September 2000. Lewis died in November 2000.

In a letter to the journal editor, Helen wrote, "My fifteen-year-old son, Lewis, died in November 2000 as a result of complications following the procedure. You may imagine my surprise when I read the opening section in the results section of this article which said, 'There were no deaths.' . . . It cannot help but raise questions . . . three of [the authors] were intimately aware of Lewis's case. For those looking for information, such omissions are fundamentally misleading. An outcome review cannot pick and choose its findings." She received a reply saying that the article would not be changed.

But the journal article did confirm that the operation Lewis had resulted in a higher complication rate, more pain, and a longer recovery time in the hospital compared with the traditional surgery. Helen says that this finding was the opposite of information publicly available on the internet and on the hospital's website, which portrayed the procedure as simpler, safer, and easier on the patient than the traditional surgery. Moreover, in a study that was supposed to be about complications of the surgery, the article failed to include the ultimate complication—death.

Helen believed that this article in a respected medical journal would put a serious damper on the enthusiasm for the new procedure. She was wrong. Four months later, on July 22, 2002, the cover story of *U.S. News & World Report*'s annual "America's Best Hospitals" issue featured the surgery Lewis had for funnel chest. The article mentioned the results of the 1998 study of forty-two children, the same article Helen had obtained from Lewis's surgeon. The *U.S. News & World Report* story did not mention any of the later findings that showed high rates of complications. It only described other minimally invasive surgeries and offered a few cautionary notes that they "can be risky because even the simplest ones are harder to do than their open equivalents. That means the procedure is harder to learn and possibly more hazardous if a surgeon hasn't done a fair number and isn't doing it regularly."

In a letter to the editor of *U.S. News & World Report*, Helen expressed her astonishment that the surgery was reported as a "shining example of low-complication minimally invasive surgery. . . . In the medical literature, the minimally invasive procedure is solidly documented as resulting in longer hospitalizations, higher costs, a higher complication rate, and significantly higher postoperative pain. On average, 20 to 25 percent of these surgeries result in complications. My fifteen-year-old son, who died of complications of the procedure, was one of the casualties of this ongoing nationwide experiment. It was glowing, unquestioning press accounts such as yours that persuaded us to subject our healthy child to this unnecessary surgery. The so-called success of the procedure lies not in consistently good surgical outcome but in shrewd marketing to the enormous pool of unsuspecting potential patients." Helen's letter was not published.

"In my view, the article in *U.S. News & World Report* was an end run around the medical literature," Helen says. "Old-fashioned medical research was no match for modern public relations."

The minimally invasive surgery continues to be performed. "Patients must be able to weigh risks and benefits," Helen says. "But the first question for the patient should be whether the surgery is necessary at all. I frankly despair over the current climate in which hospitals seem to see a need to drum up business, particularly elective surgery, rather than be a community resource that performs a service when needed.

"Pediatric surgery is not a commodity to be marketed like toothpaste. Toothpaste can't kill. Surgery can. We need to make a public issue of the biased, often evasive process that passes for medical decision-making. The unspoken code of silence on the front end is one of the fundamental problems of medicine. It leads to needless risk, needless treatment, and spiraling costs. If people had transparent information about risk, or what a surgery or treatment could actually do for them, they would probably decline a lot of the treatment that is offered."

Helen's instinct is correct. When people are fully informed, they are more likely to choose a less intensive treatment option. "A small but growing body of research is telling us that patients actually want less than we are giving them. Perhaps one way to temper our addiction to doing everything is to let patients tell us when they have had enough," says Dr. James Weinstein at the Dartmouth Medical School.

A BETTER WAY

Helen's search for the truth was relentless, even though it was too late to save her son. Without public access to information, it would have been far more difficult for her to learn about the surgery and its outcomes and complications. But not everyone can devote the time, energy, and commitment to do what Helen did. It is also not very efficient for every person contemplating a surgery or other serious medical intervention to conduct his or her own research. Why should the 250,000 people who have heart bypass surgery every year conduct their own individual research on treatment options, risks, and benefits?

Progressive leaders in medicine have concluded that physicians need a way to access available evidence so they can make better recommendations to patients. It is impossible for doctors to stay up to date on all the information about treatment options for a particular medical condition, and their benefits and risks. Patients and families—including doctors who become patients—need a similar road map to navigate the thorny thicket. The Foundation for Informed Medical Decision Making, a Boston-based nonprofit, does exactly this. With a staff of researchers and physician consultants from around the country, it reviews the science and evidence about a condition, treatment options, and the risks and benefits of each. It creates state-of-the-art DVDs with videos that include real patients who have made decisions about treatment options. The evidence from the best and most current research is woven through the patients' experiences. The foundation receives no funding from companies that make money selling products or services that have a stake in the treatment choices.

An epic battle will continue to be waged between good science and Madison Avenue marketing. Throughout the United States, new ideas and treatments are developed by people with noble intentions. Good intentions then morph into business imperatives. Good ideas are translated into real-world applications for people who can benefit. But honorable business often turns into a feverish sales pitch with all the requisite glitz. The purpose of medical care is lost in the din of the pitch.

The people on the front lines who lie down on the gurney are the forgotten ones. The only shield they have is the wisdom to know the difference between solid evidence and commercial promotion. That wisdom may come from their own due diligence or a stroke of luck in finding good people whose sole purpose is their best interest.

8 MARINATED MINDS

THINK OF BARBECUE SAUCE. Or a special homemade recipe for marinating steaks. Marinades make food more attractive and palatable. To be effective, they must be acidic. Acid destroys the boundaries of cells created by nature for protection. As the marinade permeates, the food is forever changed. It becomes malleable, or more precisely, like gelatin.

Today our minds are marinated in news, so-called news, marketing, television dramas, and internet advertising. Surgery becomes palatable, perhaps attractive. On the internet we can watch human bodies being cut open in a live broadcast of surgery. It becomes attractive to take a pill that is advertised on television—and, by the way, has side effects that can kill. Our minds have been reset to believe it's okay.

The media marinade disconnects us from the reality of what we allow others to do to our bodies. We suspend our critical thinking. We are advised, "Ask your doctor." Let others do our thinking for us, we are told. Who are we, the unschooled and unknowing, to think for ourselves?

In the marinade, new beliefs are conceived, born, nurtured, and sustained. Expectations are created. Belief begets dogma, and dogma becomes reality. Is it any wonder that almost 34 percent of Americans believe that modern medicine can cure just about anything? In contrast, only 11 percent of Germans believe this to be true. The optimism in America's genes and the can-do spirit that flows through its veins might explain this difference. Or maybe it's the marinade.

The marinade is a mixture of media-filled medical hype, miracles, makeovers, and marketing. A steady diet of it convinces us that more is always better. The United States is the only country besides New Zealand that allows pharmaceutical companies, device manufacturers, and other purveyors of health-care treatments to advertise directly to consumers.

National and local television news, magazines, newspapers, and even medical dramas on television are Trojan horses for the next press release about a big breakthrough that really isn't. Gary Schwitzer is the founder of Health News Review, a website devoted to improving the accuracy of health-care news stories. HealthNewsReview.org reviews news stories that make a therapeutic claim about treatments, procedures, drugs or devices, vitamins or nutritional supplements, and diagnostic and screening tests. It takes no money from any vested interest. A team of reviewers from the fields of journalism, medicine, health services research, and public health assesses the quality of the stories using a standardized rating system. Stories are graded, and critiques appear on the website. Stories that are accurate, balanced, and provide complete information receive a five-star rating.

Schwitzer offers a sobering assessment of the state of health-care journalism based on his own survey of health-care journalists. The findings are alarming. Just about half (44 percent) of staff journalists participating in the survey say their organization sometimes or frequently bases stories on news releases without substantial additional fact-gathering. Especially alarming is that 32 percent of journalists who responded to the survey acknowledge that their news organizations sometimes allow advertisers or sponsors to influence health-care news. "This is an amazing admission," Schwitzer says, "and perhaps the most troubling finding in the entire survey."

THE EPIDEMIC OF FAKE HEALTH-CARE NEWS

Trudy Lieberman, a veteran journalist and director of the Health and Medicine Reporting Program at the Graduate School of Journalism at City University of New York, has investigated the cozy relationships between hospitals and local television stations. Her work has uncovered how hospitals use the local media to market their services.

The local television station's health-care reporter might host a half-hour show, with the hospital paying for the airtime. More often than not, according to Lieberman, the hospital controls the story. Its personnel may even edit scripts written by station newspeople. "Viewers who think they are getting news are really getting a form of advertising," says Lieberman. Local stations across the country are less likely to report on medical mistakes or hospital-acquired infections because of this cozy atmosphere. It can be impossible for educated consumers to know the difference between real news and paid advertising aimed at attracting unsuspecting patients.

Arrangements such as these occur because local television stations want inexpensive stories that require little work, and hospitals want to attract customers. The result is an epidemic of fake health-care news, according to Lieberman. The news becomes just another way to advertise.

The seismic shift that has occurred in the blurring of lines between news and advertising is captured in the words of a veteran journalist, Clare Crawford-Mason, who reported on the White House for nearly twenty years. She quips, "It used to be that television was about bringing the news to audiences. Now it's about bringing audiences to advertisers."

When television advertising is made to look like news, it can be hard to see the difference. A smiling middle-aged man wearing a blue hospital gown is shown walking in a hospital hallway, presumably after knee-replacement surgery. This image aired in a made-for-television hospital advertisement in Philadelphia after the evening news had ended, though it had the look and feel of a news broadcast. The advertisement told viewers that if they gave the hospital twenty-four hours, it would give them new knees. Surgery was portrayed as a piece of cake—though fiddling with the knees is never simple.

The advertisement might be perceived as a public service, but the hospital has a financial interest in getting people in the door. If viewers call the telephone number on their television screen, they will not receive independent and objective information on how good the hospital is at fixing knees, or the infection rate or complication rate. Nor will the hospital let viewers know about the excruciating pain that can occur after surgery. Gary Schwitzer cautions:

"You are probably being sold a bill of goods if you are not hearing about the possible harms or how a new approach compares to an existing treatment."

THE MISSING INGREDIENT IN THE MARINADE

The marinade lacks a critical ingredient. The risks and possible harm of a test, procedure, or new device are underplayed or never reported. So most people do not know what they are getting themselves into.

Dr. Eric Holmboe and his associates wanted to know whether people understood the risks and benefits of an elective angioplasty they were having the next day. In their survey, they found that most patients were unaware of the risks. More than half the people—54 percent—could not recall a single risk. Either they were not told or did not remember being told. Twenty-five percent said they had had no conversation with their doctor about the risks, which include stroke, heart attack, and death—the very outcomes they believed the procedure could prevent. Dr. Holmboe says that many people do want information from their doctors about the risks and benefits of medical procedures.

In another study, conducted at the University of Michigan, three thousand adults over age forty who had to make a decision about a surgery, a test, or medication were asked about their conversation with their doctor beforehand. Most people did not know much about the possible complications, side effects, and risks. Their doctors were much more likely to discuss the benefits. Only 20 percent of those facing a decision about back surgery, for example, knew important facts about it, and just 30 percent of people contemplating knee-replacement or hip-replacement surgery were aware of critical information.

With the explosion of health-care information, many newly empowered individuals are sifting through internet pages to find medical care that is right for them. Many are asking for treatment they should never receive. In a *Consumer Reports* survey of 39,000 subscribers and 335 primary-care physicians, 40 percent of doctors reported that patients bring information from the internet that is inaccurate or misunderstood. Thirty percent said that patients ask for unnecessary tests.

Patients may ask for more than just unnecessary tests. Geri Amori, a former hospital risk manager in Vermont, remembers a patient who was determined to exercise her rights as a consumer. "A patient called me with complaints about two doctors. She had been scheduled for a gynecological surgery and a knee surgery. When both surgeries were canceled, she was upset." When Geri talked with the two physicians involved, they told her that they had initially agreed to perform the surgeries because the patient pressured them, but the more they thought about it, each of them wanted to try a less invasive approach.

Geri called the patient and said, "Both doctors said they scheduled the surgeries for you but believe there are better ways to take care of you." The patient replied, "That's not appropriate. I'm the customer. If I want surgery, I should get surgery. And I can pay for it. I have an insurance card." Geri reminded her, "Physicians take an oath to do no harm, and they have an ethical obligation to use the least invasive approach."

The patient said, "The issue is, I'm the customer." Geri asked, "What do you want me to do?" "I want you to make the doctors do the surgery," the patient replied. This was not about to happen, so the woman ended the conversation by asking, "Where can I have the surgery done?" Geri replied, "Not here."

Patients come to doctors with expectations derived from earlier experiences or from hearing information from advertisements or friends or family. Dr. Paul Batalden at the Dartmouth Medical School remembers the first few months of his practice as a young pediatrician. "I was seeing a little kid with a sore throat. His usual doctor was away. I examined him and found that he didn't have much of a fever, his ears were fine, and his chest was clear. He had an upper respiratory infection. I said to his mother, 'I think your son has a sore throat. I'll culture it and we'll know in twenty-four hours whether he has strep. I don't think it is, but that would be the only reason to treat him with antibiotics.'

"The mother replied, 'Aren't you going to do blood work?' I said to her, 'I don't believe blood work is needed.' The mother continued, 'His usual doctor always gets blood work.' I responded, 'I can appreciate that this might have been his practice. I really don't think we need to do that today. Tomorrow we'll know whether his throat culture is positive.' She shook her head in disbelief."

The next day the mother called and was told that the throat culture was negative. She persisted and wanted to talk to her son's regular doctor, believing that the new young doctor had not been thorough. The boy's usual doctor called the mother and prescribed antibiotics. Dr. Batalden says, "I was ready to do it right, but I was up against this prior relationship and expectations."

An episode from *Grey's Anatomy*, while fictional, highlights how young doctors in training can be thoroughly steeped in the marinade.

The ambulance pulls up in front of the hospital emergency room, sirens blaring. The paramedic jumps out and shouts to the waiting doctors, "Sixty-one-year-old male, Otis Sharon, found unconscious on the street corner with a swollen ankle." The man's vital signs are stable, and he is alert and speaking. An eager young surgery resident hollers, "He's mine."

A contest is taking place among the surgery residents at the fictional Seattle Grace Hospital. The most points will be awarded for diagnosing an underlying and unexpected medical condition in a patient. The contest winner will receive a coveted prize, and the contest will end the night of Sharon's visit to the emergency room.

Dr. Stevens, the resident who claimed Sharon as her patient, is twenty-six points behind in the contest. She tells her peers, who are wondering why she is enthused about taking care of a patient with a swollen ankle, "You see swollen ankles. I see medical mystery. Eighty points."

Once inside the emergency room, Sharon is alert and talking. Dr. Stevens asks him if has been feeling dizzy. He replies, "Maybe a little." She continues, "Have you had any recent traumas?" He quips, "I go back and forth to the East Coast for my job. Does that count?" Demurring, she asks, "Any mosquito bites?" Now Sharon is getting worried. "Do I have something bad—malaria, or West Nile virus?" She reassures him, "No need to panic. We're going to take this one step at a time."

Dr. Stevens reiterates to another resident, "I'm twenty-six points behind. . . . Eighty points to solve the medical mystery . . . the holy grail of the contest." She turns to

Sharon and says, "Is there anyone I can call? Maybe you shouldn't be alone here today." At this point Sharon has been diagnosed only with a hairline fracture in his ankle. A barrage of tests is planned. "I want to go home. I want to go home," he shouts. "I'm alone and scared in some hospital with some beautiful young doctor holding my hand . . . trying to figure out what horrible disease I'm going to die of."

Dr. Stevens performs a spinal tap and Sharon screams in pain. "It's okay," she reassures her patient. "It's not okay, it hurts . . . I'm alone and I'm not okay, I'm dying." Once again she reassures him, "I am going to find out what's wrong with you. . . . You're being given a second chance at life." She continues with the procedure. "You're going to feel a little pressure," "Ow . . . oow," he shouts in pain.

Dr. Bailey, the chief resident, appears a short time later. "Why did we do a spinal tap on an ankle fracture? . . . How many points? Don't tell me you are putting this man through painful and unnecessary procedures so you can win a contest," she asks Dr. Stevens with more than a hint of indignation. Dr. Stevens acknowledges that she does want to win the contest, but she explains that she wants to make sure the man doesn't leave the hospital with meningitis or another rare disease. Dr. Bailey replies, "All right then, carry on."

Later in the episode, Dr. Stevens is clearly disappointed with the result of the tests. An intern is standing by and asks, "Ankle guy?" Dr. Stevens rattles off the tests she has performed; all the results are normal. The intern says, "The fact is that you are doing unnecessary medical procedures to win a contest . . . Oh my God . . . Great doctors know when to stop." Dr. Stevens reiterates, "I have to win it."

The moment of truth finally arrives when Dr. Stevens tells Sharon, "Nothing bad came up." He asks, "What about all those alphabet tests?" Sheepishly she tells him, "They likely indicated that you basically have a minor flu." With undisguised anger, he shouts, "This whole day—everything you put me through—you put me through all this for the flu? . . . I wouldn't have had to go through the hell . . . You treated me like a rat, like a rat in a perverted lab. Give me my prescription. I want to get out of here." She tells him that the flu doesn't respond to antibiotics, just fluids and rest. "I'm really, really sorry," she tells him.

Dr. Stevens didn't win the contest. Another resident won the award—a pager, the holy grail of the hospital's surgery residency program. It's part of a tradition at the made-for-television hospital. The pager has been passed down over the many years the contest has been held there. The winner may assist on any surgery for three months.

While this is a fictional story, it illustrates how no one steps in to halt the runaway train of unwarranted tests. The marinade has worked. The mind of a young person in medical training has been reset, disconnected from the reality of what is done to a patient. Critical thinking is suspended; the patient as a person is invisible. The purpose of medicine is not the patient. It's something else. It's a game. And it's all about winning.

9 THE CHAPTER YOU WON'T WANT TO READ

THE GREEN MONSTER in the health-care system was born in the post–World War II era when Americans believed that anything was possible. In the heyday of optimism, the federal government authorized vast new sums of money for health care and ceded control over its use to the medical and scientific elite.

At the time, the nation had good reason to express such faith in science and medicine. On April 12, 1955, when epidemiologists at the University of Michigan announced that the Salk vaccine was successful in preventing polio, the great scourge of the time, fear was replaced by immense relief and joy. According to an account of the momentous occasion, "People observed moments of silence, rang bells, honked horns, blew factory whistles, fired salutes, kept their traffic lights red in brief periods of tribute, took the rest of the day off, closed their schools or convoked fervid assemblies therein, drank toasts, hugged children, attended church, smiled at strangers, forgave enemies." The discovery was profound, the gratitude authentic, the joy universal.

Public coffers were opened wide. The National Institutes of Health was the nation's premier biomedical research enterprise. Congress gave scientists the autonomy to set their own rules and determine research priorities that merited public funding. The NIH budget ballooned from 1955 to 1960.

Congress supported a massive program of hospital construction that in the 1950s and 1960s poured billions of dollars into congressional districts throughout the country. The money created jobs and helped reelect members of Congress. With faith in science and an insatiable desire for health, an immense new system of medical schools and teaching hospitals was created. Congress outlawed federal interference in how public money for science would be spent.

Once the infrastructure for medical research and health-care delivery was built, Americans wanted access to it. Medicare was established in 1965 along with its companion program, Medicaid, for low-income Americans and people with disabilities who need long-term care and support.

The green monster of health care had grown up and was ready to leave home. Now it has an insatiable appetite and is fattened by unfettered access to the country's refrigerator, pantry, and seed corn to grow tomorrow's food. The federal government borrows money from China to feed it. The bigger it gets, the more bold it becomes. It is oblivious to economic recession. No one has had the guts to ask it to stop, or at least to curtail its voracious appetite.

The green monster lives in all fifty states, in rural and urban areas, and among the rich and the poor. While many health-care organizations maintain high ethical standards, it nonetheless is invited into all types of health-care facilities—big hospitals and small ones, doctors' offices, ambulatory surgery centers, diagnostic imaging centers, and everywhere else. Here are examples of the green monster's creativity as told by health-care insiders.

THE MIAMI PROSTATECTOMY

A hospital chief executive officer in Florida recalls a meeting of physicians in Miami where a urologist unabashedly described the "Miami prostatectomy." This procedure is designed so that the patient gets a good flow of urine but will need another surgery in two years. None of the physicians present for the meeting challenged the ethics of treating patients in a manner that deliberately created repeat customers. The hospital CEO says, "Some areas of the country are 'obscene' in the way care is provided to patients. I was happy to get out of that part of the country."

THE DONUT SHOP

"We are like a donut shop," says a young chief operating officer to a physician at the hospital where he works. "Our job is to sell donuts. If we don't sell a lot of donuts, we go out of business. Your job, as chief of emergency services, is to convince patients they need to be in the hospital and to convince doctors they have to admit patients." So wrote a physician who responded to a survey conducted in 2007 by the American College of Physician Executives, which published the survey results, along with this comment, in its journal. The organization's members include chief medical officers and vice presidents for medical affairs at hospitals and other health-care organizations.

COLLEGE TUITION

A health-care insider describes a group of physicians who worked diligently to reduce preventable deaths among patients in their community who had undergone heart bypass surgery. In the best tradition of medicine, they studied one another's best practices and applied them. Together they saved lives. This same group of doctors knew that one of their peers in the community performed more bypass surgeries than anyone else. No one questioned him. Privately the doctors believed that the patients did not need the surgeries, but they explained his actions saying, "Oh, he's got four kids in college." When the insider was asked, 'What will it take to get this guy to stop?' the reply was, "When the kids graduate from college."

A vice president for risk management at a medical malpractice insurance company says that she has seen cases where family financial pressures may motivate doctors to increase their volume. "Our underwriter has noticed that when some physicians reach their early fifties and are facing retirement and have kids in college, they tend to increase their volume. They can't handle it, and we see malpractice cases filed."

HAVE GROIN, WILL CATH

A physician who worked in private practice described how his colleagues were eager to perform cardiac catheterizations. The mantra in the office was, "Have groin, will cath" (referring to a catheter, or long, thin tube inserted in an artery in the groin and threaded through the blood vessels to the heart). The doctor left this practice to work in the Veterans Health Administration, where doctors are paid a salary and have no financial incentive to perform unnecessary medical procedures.

LAMBORGHINIS IN THE JUNGLE

A doctor who has practiced medicine in an East Coast hospital for many years says, "When I was in training, I drove an old Chevy. The doctors who taught us drove Chevys too, but they were new. Now I look around the parking lot of our hospital and count the Lamborghinis. As far as I'm concerned, people can drive whatever car they want. But you have to ask, who is paying for it? It's a bit graphic, but overuse is like the nature programs on **PBS** television. When the tigers or lions kill their prey, all kinds of creatures come to share in the feast. This is what happens to patients. I see it every day. When a doctor admits a patient to the hospital, he might call in six, eight, or ten consultants. Each one bills the patient. No one questions whether the procedure or whatever the consulting doctors do benefits the patient. It's a feeding frenzy."

He continues. "Not far from here a group of doctors refer patients to each other. They do all sorts of things to them, and they give each other kickbacks. The patients think it is good care, but they don't know enough to know otherwise. It's not good care. It's exploitation. It's assault and battery. It happens every day in doctors' offices. The government allows the doctors to be crooks. It's a form of organized crime, and no one does anything about it."

NO CHILD LEFT BEHIND

Children are not immune from unnecessary tests and treatments. A pediatrician from Texas observed unnecessary diagnostic tests when she first started practicing medicine. "I remember a group of pediatricians here in town that would admit healthy, well-nourished children to the children's hospital and run them through a series of diagnostic tests to detect some sort of malnourishment disorder. I was told that after many years the medical director of the hospital finally ordered them to stop. Mostly, doctors can do what they want."

JUST RACKING THEM UP

A physician describes how twenty years ago a hospital on the East Coast that specializes in heart bypass surgery performed operations on people whose medical condition did not require surgery. "They had a production line and were just racking them up," he says. He estimates that 20 percent of the procedures were probably unnecessary. Today the hospital advertises on a local radio station that it performs 100,000 heart procedures a year.

THE MACHINE IS GRINDING PEOPLE UP

Another physician claims the problem of needless care is growing worse. "About ten years ago there used to be a few people doing bad medicine for money. Now, doing bad medicine for money has become institutionalized. The economic machine is grinding people up for money. The hospital where I worked used to be a friendly place to practice medicine. Five years ago the hospital decided it wanted to grow high-profit surgeries such as major vascular procedures [abdominal aneurysms, seven-hour arterial bypass surgery, etc.], thoracic cases, and complex back surgeries. They brought in god-awful surgeons, the worst I've seen in twenty years. I remember one guy who had bad hands and terrible judgment, and the mortality rate for his patients was huge when it should have been 5 percent. Another guy had tremendous complication rates but was immune from criticism because he's from a well-to-do family in the community and is on the board of the hospital.

"Every week cases are done at this hospital that shouldn't be done. And when patients die from complications of surgery that should not even be done, I call it 'white collar murder.' The worst thing is to be on a case where you are not helping someone and where the patient might be made worse off. Years ago this would happen once in a while. Now it happens all the time. Meanwhile, from the outside, the hospital looks great. The president gets awards from the chamber of commerce, and if you were a board member you would think the hospital was doing a good job. On the inside it's a different story. If you try to speak up, the administration comes after you because you are jeopardizing business. I had to quit my job and escape this hospital because I couldn't guarantee good care for my patients. I'm going to a place where I hope economics won't prevent my providing good care for them."

IF THE PUBLIC ONLY KNEW

A nationally recognized nursing leader has witnessed firsthand how hospital leaders can create a culture where overuse is sanctioned and encouraged. She worked for many years at a hospital with a CEO who supported a strict process that granted privileges only to doctors who were competent and practiced safe care. When a new CEO arrived, his agenda was to improve the hospital's bottom line, gain immediate physician support, and keep the doctors satisfied. The strict quality and safety-driven standards used for granting doctors hospital privileges were immediately downgraded. The nursing chief says, "The new CEO's approach was all about getting doctors in the door to do procedures, make money, and not anger the physician partners who were trying to get their colleagues in. This led to a measurable deterioration in the quality and safety of patient care. If the public only knew what goes on, trust would plummet to the ground."

A SPECIAL VITAMIN C

A conscientious nurse worked with a small group of physicians in a private practice in the Midwest. She recalls, "One day an older patient called, and she was crying. 'I can't afford to buy the medicine the doctor said I should take,' she said. The woman had Parkinson's disease, and the doctor had told her that the medicine could help stop the progression of the disease. The bottle of twenty pills cost $60."

The nurse asked the woman to read the information on the bottle. It said "ascorbic acid," which is Vitamin C. "I thought she was mistaken," the nurse recalls. "So I asked her to put her husband on the phone. We spoke for a few minutes, and I suggested that he come to the office with the bottle so I could look at it. Within an hour he arrived with the empty bottle of medicine. Sure enough, the label read 'ascorbic acid.' I have seen patients put pills in bottles that are not the original bottle from the pharmacy, so I asked the husband, 'Is this your wife's medicine, or is it vitamins?' He replied, 'These are her special vitamins for her Parkinson's.'" The nurse told him to take the bottle to the local pharmacy and ask for a certain pharmacist who would find the same vitamins that cost much less.

"I finally understood why the doctor never wanted me to talk to his patients. The doctor's son was selling dietary supplements, and this Vitamin C was the brand he sold. I had thought he didn't want me to take his calls because I had not proven myself, even though I took sixty calls a day for the other doctors. The truth is, he was trying to hide what he was doing." Sure enough, when the doctor returned from vacation and the nurse told him what had happened, he snapped, "How dare you talk to my patients. This is a special Vitamin C." The nurse says, "I couldn't wait to get out of there."

"I HAVE A HOUSE PAYMENT"

A hospital CEO describes how a doctor who discovers a benign cyst on a patient's back can let it go, thinking, "It's on the patient's back. It's not visible." Or he can say, "That cyst could be a problem down the road. And I have a house payment. You know, I think we ought to take it out." A good doctor will say this is a needless surgery.

"WHO IS LOOKING OUT FOR US?"

Deandra Vallier, the wife of the lawyer who had bladder surgery for nonexistent cancer, asks, "Who is looking out for us?" The answer is that hardly anyone protects the public. Rarely do federal or state regulatory agencies intervene in cases of unnecessary medical treatment. If they do, the intervention is usually sparked by concerns about fraud, not because a person's health has been placed at risk.

An exception occurred when the Alabama state medical licensure commission alleged that an oncologist had inappropriately diagnosed or treated nineteen patients. According to the state's associate counsel, William F. Addison, "The doctor diagnosed cancer and prescribed chemo when they didn't need it." The state alleged that among the people who had inappropriate cancer treatment were:

—A ninety-two-year-old woman who went to the doctor with a small lesion on her left cheek. She was never conclusively diagnosed with cancer but was treated with chemotherapy anyway. She suffered significant side effects that required her to be treated in a hospital emergency room.

—A seventy-three-year-old woman with a history of breast cancer who was diagnosed with metastatic breast cancer and treated with chemotherapy. She had a history of stroke, seizures, and diabetes. She suffered major complications from the chemotherapy that required her to be placed on a feeding tube for a period of time. According to the state, the patient did not have metastatic breast cancer; the treatment exposed her to unnecessary risk and discomfort.

—A fifty-seven-year-old woman who was diagnosed with an accelerated phase of a type of leukemia and treated aggressively with chemotherapy, which resulted in cardiac arrest. She was resuscitated. According to state records, there was no evidence that the patient needed the aggressive treatment that nearly led to her death.

The medical board sought an emergency suspension of the doctor's license. When the doctor went to court to protest, the judge stayed the suspension because the doctor had not been sued for malpractice. Two weeks after the judge's decision, a sixty-five-year-old breast cancer survivor sued the doctor. According to state records, the doctor told her that the breast cancer had returned. No biopsy was performed, yet he wrote in the patient's record that she had metastatic breast cancer that had spread to her spine. The woman sought a second opinion from Memorial Sloan-Kettering Cancer Center, where a doctor concluded that she had no evidence of recurrent breast cancer and recommended that she not continue chemotherapy. The state argued that the physician had violated a cardinal principle that one should not treat cancer without first obtaining tissue confirmation. The woman suffered emotional trauma from being told she had a fatal disease, plus the physical trauma of toxic chemotherapy. After a protracted legal battle, the state revoked the doctor's license to practice medicine.

State medical boards grant licenses to physicians and discipline those who violate the public's trust. Many members of state medical boards and their staff are conscientious and seek earnestly to protect the public, but fierce political opposition from doctors who want to maintain their licenses and autonomy at any cost sometimes prevents them from protecting the public adequately. Bowing to political pressure, state legislatures chronically underfund medical boards so they lack the money, people, and power to be guardians for the public. Americans have little protection from autonomy run amuck.

In rare instances, doctors are criminally prosecuted for providing unnecessary treatment. A Sarasota, Florida, dermatologist who performed a certain type of surgery for skin cancer was convicted in 2006 by federal prosecutors of performing unnecessary surgeries on seventy older patients he diagnosed as having skin cancer but who in fact did not have the disease. Ellen Murray was one of his patients who had had eight surgeries performed by him over seven years before she realized something was amiss. Like many patients who discover they have received unnecessary and inappropriate medical treatment, the realization occurred only after time had passed. She says, "It's still hard to accept the fact that a doctor would do unnecessary surgery for money." She became suspicious when the doctor diagnosed skin cancer once again, and she sought a second opinion that revealed no cancer.

Murray contacted the fraud hotline at the federal Centers for Medicare and Medicaid Services, which administers the Medicare program, to report the doctor's unscrupulous activities. She recalls being told that if the doctor performed the service, he or she would be reimbursed for it. Being a determined woman, Murray did not stop there.

She blew the whistle and filed a claim under the federal False Claims Act. According to the act, whistle-blowers have a financial incentive to provide information about anyone who cheats the government. The False Claims Act was enacted in 1863 during the Civil War when the Union army was sold guns that did not fire, horses that could barely walk, and bags of sawdust instead of gunpowder. President Abraham Lincoln was a strong proponent and urged Congress to pass the law, which came to be known as the Lincoln Law.

The U.S. Department of Justice joined the False Claims Act lawsuit after its investigation found that many of the doctor's patients had had unnecessary surgery for nonexistent skin cancer. The Sarasota dermatologist was convicted and was sentenced to twenty-two years in federal prison. The case illustrates that the only legal recourse for people harmed by unnecessary medical treatment is to prove fraud. The doctor was convicted of defrauding Medicare, not harming patients.

HOW CAN THIS HAPPEN

How can a doctor perform unnecessary surgery on a patient? Dr. Brad Stuart, a Stanford-trained internist, explains it this way: "The system rewards people for doing something and generating as much income as possible. We do and do, and can't stop doing. As doctors, we don't want to see the cruelty and pain we inflict on people. If we took the time to look, we would stop inflicting pain. But we don't stop to look, feel, or think. If we did, we would be paralyzed by guilt.

"The dehumanization begins in medical school. We are trained not to look at the pain we inflict, or the pain we feel when we inflict pain on others. So doctors may put their feelings to sleep and place their shame and guilt far from consciousness. Others are willing to stay awake while still others who went to sleep are willing to wake up. The moment of awakening can be horribly painful. Great physicians have either stayed awake or been willing to wake up. They feel the impact of what they do in the very core of their being."

Dr. Lucian Leape of the Harvard School of Public Health says, "It is quite obvious that the cause of the abuse and overuse is a system that rewards people for the more they do. . . . It is time to speak up. We need to start saying this in public to change the system. I think it has totally corrupted medicine. We have taken it to more logical and ludicrous extremes. It is so fundamental that I don't think we can come to grips in a major way until we change the financing system and move toward integrated care and salaried employees working in teams."

PART III

Learn and Live

10 BYPASSING THE BYPASS

"THINK OF A HAMMER and a nail," says a physician who is vice-president for medical affairs at a hospital in Louisiana. "The hammer sees everything as a nail. Some physicians think they have a hammer, and everything they see is a nail. They stop when they run out of nails, or when the family takes away the hammer."

Americans are beginning to take away the hammer. They are asserting themselves and rejecting treatment recommendations for what they believe is unnecessary heart surgery, cancer treatment, leg amputations, back surgery, hysterectomy, mastectomy, and tonsillectomy, to name a few. They have made their decisions not cavalierly but carefully. They have studied the scientific evidence published in the medical literature, consulted doctors, used common sense, and followed their instincts.

These highly empowered people are an inspiration because of their resilience and doggedness in becoming fully informed and engaged in making medically appropriate decisions that are right for them. Stories of how they did it, and their secrets of success, provide a lesson for all: don't take medicine lying down.

A RETIRED CHEMICAL ENGINEER MAKES
HIS OWN DECISION

Howard Harwell is an eighty-seven-year-old retired chemical engineer from New Hampshire. About six years ago he developed chest pain, for which his doctor prescribed medication. As the pain gradually rose, the dosage was increased.

Howard sought another opinion from a cardiologist who recommended an angiogram. It showed that the arteries in Howard's heart had considerable calcification and blockages. He then consulted several doctors, including a cardiologist in Los Angeles who recommended that he have bypass surgery. A nephew, who is a family physician, came to the same conclusion, saying, "If there was ever an ideal case for bypass surgery, yours is it."

Howard continued his research. He contacted two nationally recognized hospitals in Boston and asked about the mortality rate of bypass surgery for men of his age, and what he could expect during recovery. One hospital said, "We do more bypasses than any hospital in the region. We'll get you on the list in no time, and Medicare will even pay for the hotel bill before you are admitted." A representative from the second hospital told him, "We can get you in here right away. We collaborate with Harvard," leading Howard to conclude that this hospital was on the cutting edge of care.

As an engineer, Howard had been trained to get all the facts before making a decision. He continued his fact-finding mission and consulted with a leading heart surgeon in New Hampshire, who asked about his situation and daily life. The doctor listened carefully. He said candidly, "In your situation, with surgery, we can make you more comfortable, but we can't offer you increased life expectancy. It's important to weigh the gain you may get in your lifestyle from surgery and compare it to the trauma of the operation. You seem to be getting along okay."

The surgeon described how it had taken a long time for the calcification to build up in Howard's heart, and how auxiliary blood vessels had probably developed to carry blood to the heart and supplement the function of the main arteries. If that were not the case, the doctor told Howard, he would probably not be alive.

The last stop in Howard's fact-finding mission was a visit to his primary-care physician. In a long conversation the doctor described his own father who, at the age of seventy-nine, had had bypass surgery and was dead in three years. "Listening to how you are getting along, and what you can and cannot do, it doesn't seem there is much you cannot do. I wouldn't recommend surgery. In fact, I recommend against it."

In the back of his mind, Howard thought of three men he knew, all about the same age, who had had bypass surgery. All three men were dead within a year of the surgery. He was also acutely aware that some people who undergo bypass surgery can suffer cognitive deficits after the surgery.

Now Howard had collected enough information to make a decision that was right for him. Other people might make a different decision with the same information. In his case, "I decided to bypass the bypass." Two years after his decision, Howard says, "I am still able to do the things

I enjoy. I'm going to play golf tomorrow, but I'll take a cart instead of walking. I ride my exercise bike every day, and I work in the garden."

What advice does Howard have for others? "It is not a good idea to delegate our health management to any doctor," he says. "I have been preaching to my wife that we have to manage our own health—do background reading and apply judgment." When Howard was asked about the enthusiasm of the two hospitals in Boston to perform surgery on him, he says, "I was a bit taken aback by the eagerness with which the hospitals wanted to take me."

Howard's fact-finding process has lessons for people facing decisions that do not require immediate action and who have time to learn and understand their options. The doctors who initially recommended that he have bypass surgery did not provide him with scientific evidence from the medical literature on the benefits and risks of the procedure. It was not until Howard found the New Hampshire heart surgeon that he learned that with his condition, bypass surgery was not likely to extend his life. Until this time, no one had informed him of this fact.

The New Hampshire heart surgeon also helped Howard think about the impact of the surgery on his life. To this point, doctors talked with Howard about the surgery, but they didn't talk about *him*. They did not discuss his quality of life and the impact the surgery might have on it. With this information, Howard could weigh the benefits and risks of bypass surgery. Ultimately he determined that for him, the risks outweighed the benefits. He was fortunate to find people who could help him make this important decision.

Just because surgery *can* be performed does not mean it *should* be performed. Howard wanted more from physicians than their informed opinions. He wanted evidence and facts so that he could weigh them and judge whether the benefits would be worth the risk.

People—both physicians and patients—have varying beliefs about medical care. Some patients are avid users of the health-care system, others stay away as much as they can. People calculate and tolerate risk differently. Life experiences and family circumstances affect beliefs and perceptions of risk. All these factors should be part of a decision to have a potentially life-altering surgery such as a heart bypass.

Not all people want to be as involved as Howard was in reaching a decision about surgery. Says Dr. Tom Delbanco, a professor at Harvard Medical School, "I can have a captain of industry who has a Harvard MBA and oversees a multi-billion-dollar company who says to me, 'Don't give me shared decision-making. Tell me what to do.' Then I can get a high school dropout in tattered jeans who saunters in my office saying, 'I want your opinion and four others, and then I'll read the internet before I decide.' I can't predict what patients will want. One of my favorite questions to a new patient is, 'What do you want your doctor to be like?'" When patients have a physician who asks a question like this, chances are they have found a good doctor who will help them make a decision that is best for them.

THE FAMILY OF A NEW YORK CITY POLICE OFFICER PUTS THEIR FOOT DOWN

Ed Lotti spent his career as a New York City police officer. A veteran of World War II, he served in the Marine Corps, fought on Okinawa, and was awarded a Purple Heart. Ed's daughter, Louise, remembers her dad lovingly and says, "My dad looked just like Archie Bunker, with his white hair and sparkly blue eyes. He was a curmudgeon just like Archie, and in fact our house looked just like Archie Bunker's house in Queens."

Ed grew up in a generation when smoking was advertised as glamorous, and he became hooked on unfiltered cigarettes. He paid little attention to his diet or his general health. After he retired from the police force at age fifty-five, he developed diabetes and suffered small strokes. When his toes showed signs of gangrene—dead tissue—he was admitted to a hospital in Queens where a surgeon removed four of his toes and part of his foot, leaving his big toe intact. After the surgery, Louise says, "Dad could still walk, thank God."

People with diabetes are more prone to foot problems because the disease can damage blood vessels and deaden nerves, resulting in a loss of sensation in the feet. Even simple blisters caused by tight-fitting shoes may trigger a decline. If gangrene sets in, doctors may have to amputate to save the person's life.

Soon after his foot surgery the doctor told Ed that he needed to have his leg amputated. "We were horrified at the thought of Dad losing his leg," Louise says. Serendipitously, a friend of hers suggested that she call a podiatrist who specialized in treating patients with foot conditions caused by diabetes. Louise was forever grateful for the advice. "The doctor took my call on a Saturday and said he would go to the hospital the next morning to see dad. We were so grateful that he took time to do this, and thank God he did. He wanted to transfer my dad to another hospital, and dad's surgeon was against it. 'You can't just take my patient out of here,' Louise recalls him saying. The podiatrist transferred him anyway, arranged a private room to ward off infection, and gave my dad a higher dose of antibiotics. This wonderful doctor saved my dad's leg. I can't tell you how much that meant to my father and our family."

During the transfer to the other hospital, Louise's mother was apprehensive and not keen about rejecting the surgeon's recommendation. Louise says, "My mom was part of the generation that didn't question or challenge a doctor. She thought a doctor is a doctor." Her mother was reassured when, as her husband was leaving the hospital in a wheelchair, she asked the nurse, "Are we doing the right thing by taking my husband to another hospital?" Louise recalls the nurse saying, "I could get fired for saying this, but you are doing the right thing."

Louise says about her dad, "When my father died a few years later at age sixty-four, he had both his legs. From the bottom of our hearts, we will be always grateful to the podiatrist."

Louise's father was fortunate. He avoided joining the ranks of more than eighty thousand Americans each year who have part of a leg amputated because of diabetes. Good foot care can prevent most diabetes-related amputations. The lesson from Ed's story is what many families have come to realize: a person who becomes a patient sometimes needs help in advocating for proper care. For many families, going against a doctor's recommendation is uncharted territory. It some cases it is the right thing to do.

A WHITE HOUSE CORRESPONDENT REFUSES SURGERY

"I am your ultimate pain-in-the-ass patient," Clare says. This former journalist and senior producer for NBC News says, "I have a healthy skepticism of all authority. In fact I once had a doctor who fired me as his patient. He wanted to x-ray anything that moved, and I refused. I have successfully avoided all surgery since I had my tonsils taken out when I was six years old. Chances are that wasn't necessary either."

Not long ago, doctors set wheels in motion for Clare to have a hysterectomy. While taking a small daily dose of estrogen to curb the symptoms of menopause, she also had biannual biopsies to detect possible uterine cancer. When one lab report showed atypical cells in her uterus, her doctor said this finding indicated cancer and recommended a hysterectomy. At age sixty-five, Clare was on the road to joining millions of American women who have had their uteruses surgically removed.

As a veteran journalist, Clare knows how to dig for the truth, so she started digging. She obtained opinions from three more doctors. One doctor reviewed the lab report and concluded that a hysterectomy was her only alternative. Clare's internist came to the same conclusion. "The doctors suggested that I could prevent the possibility of ovarian cancer if they removed my ovaries while they were in there taking out my uterus," Clare said. "I got the feeling that after menopause, a woman's reproductive parts are a liability."

The third doctor, a physician from Johns Hopkins who read the lab report, said Clare had a 25 percent chance of having cancer already and that a hysterectomy was warranted. She asked him if he would read the biopsy slide that showed the abnormal cells. He agreed to do so and to have a leading pathologist read it with him. Clare realized that while all the physicians who recommended surgery had read the lab report, none had read the biopsy slide itself. Until this point, the only person who had read the slide was the technician who wrote the lab report.

Without much hope for a reprieve from surgery, Clare prepared herself. She made a living will and authorized a power of attorney. She rearranged her house so she would not have to climb the stairs to her bedroom. To be ready for any eventuality, she received the last rites of the Catholic church. As the day of surgery approached, she still had not heard from the physician who had agreed two weeks earlier to read the biopsy slide.

Clare had once worked with W. Edwards Deming, an internationally renowned statistician who taught business leaders how to improve the quality of their products and services. After World War II, General Douglas MacArthur had invited Deming to Japan to teach industrial leaders methods of quality control and principles of management. Today Deming is regarded in Japan as the father of the country's postwar industrial revitalization. His principles underpin the global success of companies such as Toyota.

Clare had produced an NBC television program that introduced American viewers to Deming's ideas of quality management. She had also interviewed him for a library of videos and two books about his teachings.

Fewer than twenty-four hours before surgery, Clare thought about the advice that Deming, who died in 1993, might have given her. He had espoused fourteen principles of management, and the fifth principle exhorted businesses to search continually for problems in order to improve every activity. Clare could hear Deming say, "Would you make a decision as important as this with a single data point, with just one person reading one slide?"

Clare knew what she needed to do. She called the physician from Johns Hopkins who had promised to read the biopsy slide. He called her back and left a message on her answering machine: "Don't have a hysterectomy unless you want one. That slide was overread."

Clare ducked the hysterectomy. Instead, the next day she had a D&C (dilation and curettage), a procedure that involves scraping and collecting tissue from the inside of the uterus. A biopsy of the cells showed no signs of cancer. Clare says, "I was saved from unnecessary surgery."

This was not the first time doctors had recommended that Clare have a hysterectomy. "When I had fibroids in the 1980s, my doctor suggested a hysterectomy," she recalls. "I asked him, 'Don't fibroids go away with menopause?' He said, 'Yes,' and since I was on the brink of it, I decided to keep my uterus—until, of course, they tried to remove it again."

The lesson from Clare's story is that patients and families are the only constant presence in the constellation of health-care professionals who come and go in the course of diagnosis and treatment. Being the constant presence, they need to make connections between discrete events. In Clare's case, the doctors saw only a series of single events: the biopsy slide, the probability of cancer, and the possibility of a lawsuit if they missed it. She saw all the dots and had to connect them. And Clare found that doctors may not question the work of their colleagues and others in the system. As she says, "That was the biggest threat to my health. I had to do that part."

A CLOSE ENCOUNTER WITH THE BUSINESS OF HEALTH CARE

Shelly is an Iowa native and a forty-two-year-old mother of two daughters. She trained to be a schoolteacher and later worked as a pharmaceutical representative. She is savvy and understands the business of health care. Her ob-gyn in a three-physician office practice in her hometown diagnosed uterine fibroids. The doctor told her that her only option was a laparoscopic hysterectomy.

Shelly describes what happened next. "I didn't want a hysterectomy, so I asked about less invasive methods that would leave my uterus intact and get rid of the fibroids. The doctor made fun of me, repeating 'less invasive methods' mockingly. Then she said, 'When that fibroid grows up over your belly button, you'll come running back!' I asked her whether my ovaries and cervix would remain, and she said, 'Well, I guess we could leave them.'" Shelly was indignant that anyone would remove perfectly healthy organs. She thought to herself, "My ovaries and cervix are perfectly fine!"

Not satisfied, Shelly saw another doctor in the practice who came to the same conclusion. Laparoscopic hysterectomy. So did the third doctor in the same practice.

"I wanted them to know that I'm not the average cabbage that fell out of the truck, so I asked for a copy of my medical records and the ultrasound so I could search for less drastic alternatives. They said, 'We only give records to our obstetric patients.' I was floored." Shelly knows that patients have a right to a copy of their medical records. When she called her insurance company to find out how the doctor's office could withhold her medical records, the company representative put her in touch with the state medical licensing board, which gives doctors their license to practice medicine. Shelly spoke to a representative of the licensing board. "I don't know what this person did," she says, "but within a day I had my records."

In the records she saw that the second doctor had written that she spent forty-five minutes discussing treatment alternatives to laparoscopic hysterectomy. "That was a lie," Shelly says. "She spent ten to fifteen minutes with me and didn't tell me about my options. That's because it would be money out of their pocket if I chose an alternative treatment that these doctors *didn't* do. All they did was laparoscopic hysterectomies, so that's what they recommended. I think it's a conflict of interest for them to steer people toward certain procedures because that's what they know and that's how they make money."

Shelly thoroughly researched treatment options and found a less drastic alternative that she believed was best for her. Her uterus is intact, and she is pleased with the results. "It's not enough for patients to know treatment options and their risks and benefits," she says. "You have to understand the business of health care." Because Shelly had worked in health care, she understood that she was led down a treatment path that might be good for the doctors' business but not for her. When asked what happens to people who don't have the skills she has, she quips, "They will have everything ripped out."

JOAN, A CANCER SURVIVOR WHO FOUND HELP FROM SPECIAL FRIENDS

"While at dinner on a Friday evening with friends, I had a pain in my chest and my head," says Joan, a long-term survivor of Hodgkin's disease, a cancer of the lymph nodes. "I said to one of my friends, 'You need to take me to the emergency room.' I thought I was having a heart attack."

In the emergency room she was greatly relieved when the physician examined her. "He knew what I was thinking, which was the worst," she says. "With a reassuring voice he said, 'You haven't had a heart attack. You are in atrial fibrillation. There is nothing medically to suggest you are in imminent danger.'" Atrial fibrillation occurs when the heart is quivering rather than beating normally.

His reassurance that she was not about to die was exactly what Joan needed: "I will never forget how much better the doctor made me feel." He discussed her heart condition and its possible link with her medical history as a survivor of Hodgkin's disease. "I don't know if the heart condition is because you are sixty years old or because of the radiation you had for the Hodgkin's disease," he explained. "People who have studied this would know. I have not studied it. I'm going to have a cardiologist come look at you."

It was ten o'clock on a Friday night when the cardiologist arrived and looked at Joan's chart. He said, "I see you had radiation to your heart thirty-five years ago. This is very serious." She remembers how he said it with such authority. "I was terrified, and I am not a terribly neurotic person." The cardiologist said she could go home, but she must see him in his office on Monday.

"I didn't sleep over the weekend because I thought I was going to die," says Joan. "As soon as I got home, I went online to the Association of Cancer Online Resources (ACOR) and found people who had had radiation for Hodgkin's disease, and it was incredibly reassuring. Other people may have gone home and had a heart attack because of fear."

Joan speaks candidly of fear, the heart-pounding, mind-numbing, gut-wrenching emotion that can take over a person's life. "Everything the first doctor did to heal my fears, the second one instilled fears I didn't even know I had. It is a paralyzing fear that keeps people from going back to the doctor. He literally left me frozen. I believe his goal was to get me so scared that I would come back three days later. I felt I was part of a quota he needed to fill on Monday and he had to close the deal—sell so many cars by the end of the month, and I was another car. I felt railroaded, sold something. It was horrible. And who knows how many tests and everything else he would have done? This happens every twenty minutes—no, every ten minutes—in doctors' offices all over the country. It is a travesty.

"I didn't go back to see the cardiologist because he left me with nothing but fear. Why would I see someone who is scary to me? He took away what I needed to trust him. This kind of person does not belong in medicine. I don't know how people like this get a license to practice."

Out of fear, most people will do what an authority figure tells them to do. Bob Davis, a former medical reporter for *USA Today*, was an emergency medical technician before becoming a journalist. While working as a reporter, he explained it this way: "We're suckers because we're scared."

Because Joan is especially resourceful, she did not simply accept what the cardiologist told her to do. "I am a sophisticated consumer. Most cardiologists do not know how to treat patients who have had Hodgkin's disease because there are not very many of us. I could tell that this cardiologist did not know what he was talking about," she says.

On Monday morning Joan went to her internist, who referred her to a different cardiologist. It was a completely different experience. Joan remembers the cardiologist saying to her, "I have seen only two people with radiation damage to the heart, and they have been very successfully treated. I'm not an expert. We'll have to run tests that anyone would run, and then you'll have to see a specialist. I would rely on you to find someone because you are very well connected in the field and would know best who they are." Joan found the best experts in the country from other patients through ACOR and made an appointment at a university hospital that treats many patients with a medical history similar to hers. She feels confident that she received the best care possible.

The lesson from Joan's experience is that when we stand on the shoulders of others, we can see more clearly. This is exactly what she did. Obtaining good health care in the twenty-first century requires people and their families to network with others who are knowledgeable and experienced and who can be lights along a dark road.

A CASE OF TRUMPED-UP AIRPLANE EAR

At Seattle-Tacoma airport on August 10, 2006, Judith and her husband, Blan, were embarking on a transcontinental journey to their home in Raleigh, North Carolina. That day, air travel in the United States had ground to a snarl. British security officials had foiled a terrorist plot to blow up as many as ten U.S.-bound airplanes with peroxide-based liquid explosives tucked into carry-on bags. Heightened security in the United States and Britain prompted mammoth delays and long lines that snaked through airports in both countries.

The infamous ban on liquids and gels in carry-on baggage had begun. Toothpaste, shampoo, contact lens cleaner, and liquid medicines were banned and tossed into giant trash bins. Judith had a long-standing sinus problem, and she packed her decongestant in checked baggage. During the long journey she became congested, and the pain in her head worsened. "The pain was killing me," she said.

When she arrived home she went to a doctor who immediately ushered her into a room where an audiologist tested her hearing. After the test she was told, "We have a brand-new hearing aid that can help you." Not to be hoodwinked, Judith walked out. She and her husband concluded that she had "airplane ear," a common condition among people who have a cold or sinus problem and travel by plane. Rapid changes in altitude and air pressure cause discomfort in the middle ear. Decongestant nasal sprays, oral decongestants, or oral antihistamines can treat it. The cost is less than five dollars. A hearing aid can cost thousands of dollars.

MARIAN, A WISE CHILD WHO PROTESTED A TONSILLECTOMY

Even at a young age, children can successfully fend off an impending surgery. Marian, a writer and editor, remembers that when she was seven years old and living in New York City, "I had frequent sore throats. Very frequent. My father also had them, and a problem with adenoids too. My parents decided, based on a recommendation from an ear, nose, and throat specialist, that I should have my tonsils taken out and that my father should as well, and his adenoids to boot. They agreed that he and I should have our procedures at the same time in order to ease any fears I might have about going to the hospital.

"A few days before the scheduled procedures, the world's chief expert on all matters, my older brother, gave me the full description of how doctors remove tonsils. They screw your head off, he said. They reach down into your throat, grab the tonsils, and yank them out. Then they screw your head back on. I was terrified, and I began pleading with my parents to allow me to skip the entire experience.

"I have no recollection of what happened next, but I still have my tonsils. I do recall that while I was in college I developed a very nasty infection in my throat. I went to the same ear, nose, and throat specialist who had operated on my father and who had been scheduled to remove *my* tonsils. While I waited in the examination room, I became curious about that earlier incident. I got out of the chair and removed my chart from the box on the door. I read about my exam at the age of seven, the recommendation for a tonsillectomy, the date of the proposed procedure, and then the following note: 'Marian's mother called. Marian has her arms and legs wrapped around the piano leg and cannot be dislodged. She REFUSES to have her tonsils removed.'

"I will always be grateful to my brother, who is today a physician, for saving me from this unnecessary procedure. But I do hope he has gotten a bit more up-to-date information on how tonsils are actually removed."

In the 1960s and 1970s, tonsillectomies were performed much more frequently than they are today. Now 80 percent fewer children have tonsillectomies than they did in 1970 because doctors concluded that the risks did not justify the benefits. Marian was ahead of her time.

ART, A NEWPAPER COLUMNIST WHO ADDED LIFE TO YEARS

At eighty years of age, Art Buchwald had a distinguished career as a humorist and syndicated newspaper columnist with the *Washington Post*. The son of a curtain manufacturer who grew up in foster homes and joined the Marines, the Pulitzer Prize–winner wrote eight thousand columns over his lifetime and more than thirty books.

Buchwald suffered from diabetes and eventually lost a leg below the knee. "Gangrene set in. . . . They took my leg, and I was furious," he said. In his newspaper columns he told his faithful readers about his later decision to forgo kidney dialysis, which would have performed the functions that his kidney no longer could and extend his life. In an interview with Diane Rehm on National Public Radio, Buchwald said, "That's the one they like you to take. They talk you into it . . . the dialysis—have to go three times a week. . . . Unless you are a certain type of person, it's not that interesting for me. . . . I finally said, 'This is not for me. I'm going the other way.' Some people objected strongly, some because they didn't want me to go. My children didn't want me to go. But they were decisions I made. . . . I'm very happy with my choices. I'm at peace with myself."

Buchwald spent what he thought would be his final weeks at a hospice in a tree-lined Washington neighborhood. He began hospice care on February 7, 2006. Against all predictions, he continued to live. "Death is on hold," he said. After five months he left the hospice, and in the summer of 2006 he went to his home on Martha's Vineyard, greeting visitors, conducting interviews, and writing another book, *Too Soon to Say Goodbye*. In his interview with Diane Rehm, he said his kidney was working. "I'm having a love affair with my kidney, and I bless him every day. . . . Some people bless their hearts . . ."

"When I decided to make my choice, it's been the happiest years of all," Buchwald told the PBS NewsHour. "I've seen friends, caught up with all the people in my life from every different place. I've been talking to people. We talk about everything under the sun." Art Buchwald died on his own terms on January 17, 2007, in Washington.

11 DO IT WITH ME, NOT TO ME

A LONGTIME CANCER SURVIVOR once said, "We're always racing for the cure. We're not racing for the care. The caring is orphan to the cure."

The stories that follow are about people who found the caring in health care. They found an oasis in an otherwise confusing and frightening landscape, a place where they were seen as a person, not as a disease. It was a place where relationships were formed and where healing could begin.

HAROLD, A NAVY VETERAN FROM NEW ENGLAND

"That son of a bitch did a PSA test," says Harold, a seventy-six-year-old navy veteran. "He snuck it in. And now I'm all worried."

Harold was talking about a doctor he went to see for a bout of bronchitis. The doctor did a PSA test without asking Harold if he wanted it. This is a blood test that measures the level of prostate-specific antigen (PSA), a protein produced by prostate cells. A PSA is often higher in men who have prostate cancer, though an elevated level of PSA does not necessarily indicate that cancer is present. The result of Harold's PSA test showed a slightly to moderately elevated level.

Harold knew he hadn't wanted a PSA test because his usual physician, Dr. Nancy Cochran, an internist at the VA Medical Center in White River Junction, Vermont, had already talked to him about it earlier that year. "Would you like to have a PSA test?" she had asked him. "Doc, I'll let you decide," Harold told her. "I'd rather that you and I make this decision together," she replied. "I have a videotape that describes the pros and cons of the test. Why don't you watch it and tell me what you think?" He agreed.

The video was produced by the Foundation for Informed Medical Decision Making, the Boston-based nonprofit. In the video, real patients talk about their decisions to have or not have a PSA test. The latest medical evidence is woven through the patients' stories. After watching the video, according to his doctor, Harold was resolute. "I don't want that test. It's not for me. Not at all."

The PSA test has been shown to detect early prostate cancer. In most cases, prostate cancer grows so slowly that most men with early evidence of the disease eventually die of something else, according to the U.S. Preventive Services Task Force, a group of health experts who review medical literature and make recommendations based on the evidence. The American Cancer Society recommends that the PSA test be offered annually, beginning at age fifty, to men who have at least a ten-year life expectancy. Older men who are likely to live less than ten years have a very small chance of benefiting from PSA screening.

At the VA Medical Center in San Francisco, researchers studied PSA screening in nearly 600,000 veterans over age 70 who receive their care at VA facilities. They wanted to know how many of these men had PSA tests performed. They found that 36 percent of men over age 85 who were seen at VA facilities and who did not have a history of prostate cancer or symptoms were given the PSA test. Fifty-six percent of men over age 70 had the test. Their findings were reported in the *Journal of the American Medical Association*.

The authors concluded that PSA screening rates among elderly veterans were too high. They were being exposed to the adverse effects of screening, including additional procedures, distress, or treatments that may result in incontinence, impotence, hip fractures, and even death. For these reasons, the authors recommended that PSA screening rates among veterans over age seventy "should be much lower than the current practice, given the known harms of screening."

For Harold, the deed had been done. Because the test result showed a slightly to moderately elevated level, he had to decide whether to have a biopsy. Dr. Cochran said to him, "You're angry that he did the test, aren't you?" "You better believe it," was Harold's reply. She reassured him, "You don't need to have the biopsy if you don't want it." Harold was enormously relieved.

If Harold had agreed to a biopsy, he would have been exposed to the risk of bleeding and infection. The biopsy might have shown a small cancer that would never become life threatening. If it did show a larger cancer, he would have to make another decision about whether to have surgery or radiation treatment.

Dr. Cochran had seen this parade of tests and treatment before. "When I was in training, I remember older men who were screened and treated for prostate cancer and suffered terrible consequences. One patient was incontinent for the remainder of his life. Another patient had chronic bleeding and required transfusions for as long as he lived. The negative consequences of treatment were underplayed."

Harold is especially fortunate to have a doctor eager to help patients make treatment decisions that are right for them. Dr. Cochran says, "Helping people make informed decisions that are right for them is the best part of medicine."

MARY, A MICROBIOLOGY TEACHER FROM NEW HAMPSHIRE

"When I did yoga, I noticed a bulge in my abdomen," says Mary, a fifty-two-year-old microbiologist from New Hampshire. She went to see a gynecologist who was affiliated with the hospital where she worked in a lab. Mary was not surprised by the diagnosis, but she was shocked by the doctor's response.

"You have uterine fibroids," Mary recalls the doctor saying. "We shouldn't wait to get them out. We can do a hysterectomy. You don't want to have any more children, so you don't need your uterus. It's a piece of cake, and women thank me afterward."

Not prepared for this sort of slam-dunk, "here's what you have to do" response from her doctor, Mary thought to herself, "Oh my gosh, this is going way too fast." She didn't have the gumption to tell the doctor that she was not ready for a hysterectomy. "I am usually assertive, but when talking to a doctor it's different." Mary mustered the courage to say, "I have no pain or bleeding. Are there alternatives?" The doctor shot back, "Why do you want to know any alternatives? You get the ultrasound and we'll set a date for the surgery. Take a look at your calendar." Mary persisted. She asked about a myomectomy, to remove the fibroids but leave the uterus intact. "Your uterus will be like Swiss cheese," was the reply.

As she left the doctor's office and walked to the parking lot, Mary knew she would not go back to this doctor. "I didn't trust her. It seemed as if she was pushing a hysterectomy because that's what she knew how to do and how she made money. I thought a female gynecologist would be more sensitive because she has the same organs in her body, but that wasn't true."

A month later Mary made an appointment with another gynecologist who also suggested a hysterectomy but said, "It sounds as if you are not ready for it. Let's do some watchful waiting." Mary burst into tears in the exam room. It was the first time a doctor had acknowledged what was important to *her*. She needed time to think.

Mary's husband of twenty-five years, a computer programmer, searched the internet for treatment options for fibroids. He read about uterine artery embolization, or UAE, a procedure that cuts off the blood supply that nourishes the fibroids. That same week Mary was at the Dartmouth-Hitchcock Medical Center in Hanover, New Hampshire, when she saw a sign, "Center for Shared Decision Making." Intrigued, Mary walked in and found a brochure about the mission of this center and brought it home to read. The next day she called and spoke to Kate Clay, its program director. "Now, I'm not going to give you advice over the phone," she remembers Kate telling her. "I'm going to send you a video about treatment options for uterine fibroids, and if you have any more questions, we can set up an appointment." The video was developed by the Foundation for Informed Medical Decision Making, the same group that developed the PSA video.

Mary and her husband watched the video the next evening at home. Four women described the options they chose to treat their fibroids and the reason for their choice. "My husband and I just looked at each other with such relief. It was so good to know that each woman had made the choice of treatment on her own terms, based on what was right for her. I felt as if a huge burden had been lifted from my shoulders. I knew the decision I needed to make. I didn't need a hysterectomy and felt confident to go against the recommendations of my family doctor and two gynecologists who all cast their vote for hysterectomy. I no longer felt as if I was backed into a corner."

Wanting to learn more about uterine artery embolization, Mary made an appointment with an interventional radiologist. He explained how UAE works and described the risks, which include infection and blood clots. Mary grew confident that UAE was the best choice for her, but she also knew that it was not a full guarantee.

"The treatment worked, and I feel great," she says with a sense of relief. "It was exhilarating to know that I could make a decision that was right for me. It was invaluable to have unbiased information about alternative treatments from a third party who didn't have a financial stake in any of the treatment options."

A NINETY-SIX-YEAR-OLD WOMAN FROM TENNESSEE

Nurses often have a good understanding of patients' wishes because they spend more time with them than any other health-care professional. Debbi, a nurse in Chattanooga, Tennessee, remembers a ninety-six-year-old woman who was admitted to the hospital from a nursing home. She had diabetes, and one of her toes was gangrenous. If it was not amputated, she would become septic and succumb to it. She was scheduled for surgery; Debbi had to obtain her consent.

"People thought she had dementia because she didn't respond when they talked to her," Debbi says. "She didn't have dementia. She was hard of hearing, and you had to talk loudly. I explained the surgery to her, and she said, 'I'm not doing that. I came into this world with all my parts, and I'm leaving with all my parts.' I said to her, 'Now, do you know what that means?' She said, 'I know what it means. I'm ninety-six years old. It's okay.' The woman was lucid and kept shaking her head, 'No, you aren't going to do that.'"

Debbi called the surgeon and told him that the operation was canceled. He wasn't very happy. Debbi said to him, "Go in and talk to her, but speak loudly so she can hear you." He came back later and popped in the door and said to Debbi, "Thank you so much."

Debbi understands that when people are facing illness, they want to be seen as the person they are, not the disease or medical condition they have. When the person is invisible and unseen, what's important to them is never known. "This patient was on the surgical train headed for the operating room. I helped her pull the emergency brake so she could get off," Debbi says. "It takes listening. Two weeks later I saw her obituary in the local newspaper. She died with all her parts, just like she wanted. Instead of looking at her as a gangrenous foot, we looked at her as a person."

A common theme can be found in the stories of Harold, Mary, and the woman from Tennessee. Each of them found a caring and knowledgeable person who helped them make an informed choice. When they were fully informed, they chose an approach that was less than what doctors were offering them. Researchers have shown that when patients are informed about their treatment options, they are more likely to choose a less intensive approach and to disagree with a doctor's recommendation for a more invasive approach. When researchers studied people with heart disease who were possible candidates for surgery, 52 percent of those who went through a learning process to be fully informed about their options chose alternatives to surgery; 66 percent of people who did not have a formal opportunity to learn about their options agreed to surgery. No apparent differences in quality of life were found between the two groups. The lesson is: knowledge is power. Another lesson: less may be more.

INFORMED CHOICE OR INFORMED CONSENT

The approach that Harold, Mary, and the woman from Tennessee used to make a decision is different from traditional informed consent. Consent is defined as when a person agrees to an action proposed by a person in a position of authority. None of these people consented to what anyone told them. They made an informed choice. A fully informed choice was possible because their medical condition was not an emergency and options were available and explained to them.

For the ninety-six-year-old woman in the hospital, the nurse initially sought her consent for surgery to remove her gangrenous toe. Instead of simply consenting to the procedure, the patient made an informed choice that was consistent with her wishes. Fortunately a conscientious nurse took the time to explain the consequences of the woman's decision to ensure that she understood. The nurse listened to her wishes and helped the physician understand the woman's preference.

Mary's first doctor steered her toward a hysterectomy. Mary felt that the doctor was making the decision for her, a decision that was inconsistent with Mary's instincts about the best course of action. In Harold's situation, the doctor who performed the PSA test did not inform him. There was no informed consent and surely no informed choice.

In the twenty-first century, many patients want greater participation in decisions about their health care. While they are not experts in medical decision-making, they do know what is important to them and their life. Not everyone wants to be deeply involved in making decisions, but informed choice will appeal to many people as the volume of information about health care increases geometrically.

WHAT A GOOD DOCTOR DOES

Every day all across the country, good doctors use their best skill and judgment and combine it with the best knowledge and evidence available to render proper care. Here is what good care from a primary-care physician looks like.

Dr. Laurence Gardner is an internist in Miami who takes pride in providing care to his patients, no more and no less than they need. When asked about how a primary-care physician prevents patients from receiving unnecessary treatment, he told this story.

"One of my patients, whom I've known for ten years, came to see me. He is seventy-six years old, very intelligent and very active. He noticed a lump on his neck, and after about three days he called for an appointment. I saw him within a week. The patient had an enlarged lymph node, so I ordered a chest x-ray to check for cancer and a blood count to check for infection. The visit lasted about fifteen minutes, and we agreed to talk in a week. The chest x-ray showed nothing, the blood count was normal."

Dr. Gardner describes what happened next, and, more important, what did not happen. "When we talked after a week, the gentleman said he thought the lump had become a little smaller. I said to him, 'Good, let's talk in another week, and I'll see you in about three weeks.' In three weeks the lymph node was one-fifth the size it had been, and it looked normal. We planned another visit in six months." In the end, the patient was fine.

What would have happened if the patient had not had a primary-care physician who practices conservative medicine? Dr. Gardner says that patients don't "stand a chance." His patient would have gone "to a specialist, probably a surgeon, hematologist, or oncologist. Expensive diagnostic tests and a biopsy would have been performed. The surgeon would have said to the patient, 'Look I'm not sure what it is, so it is better if we take it out.' The patient would have had surgery, and afterward the surgeon would have said, 'I have really good news. There was no cancer. It looks like it was just an inflammation.'"

About forty years ago Dr. Marcus Welby, a general practitioner in a suburban office, was the most popular fictional doctor on television. Known for his long-term relationships with many of his patients, who had conditions ranging from tumors to autism and addictions, he was a doctor whose qualities were appealing to many viewers. Fast forward thirty years to *Grey's Anatomy*, which features surgeons in training who perform dramatic feats. In one episode a surgery resident helps a man injured in a ferry accident who is pinned under a car. The only way to save his life is to drill small holes in his skull to relieve pressure on his brain. The resident saves his life and becomes a self-described "rock star."

From the time Dr. Welby was beamed into the homes of millions of television viewers to the first *Grey's Anatomy* episode, the number of physicians becoming sub-specialists has increased dramatically. Meanwhile the number of primary-care physicians has been plummeting. Only 20 to 25 percent of residents in internal medicine are choosing to become primary-care physicians, a precipitous drop from 54 percent a decade ago. The financial rewards of specialty medicine are seductive. If current trends continue, Americans won't be able to find a Dr. Welby in their community.

Dr. Gardner says he billed Medicare $80 for the first visit of his patient with the enlarged lymph node. It lasted fifteen minutes, and Medicare paid $40 to $50 to his practice. In the end, Dr. Gardner himself was paid less than $30. He says, "I am paid for the time I spent with the patient. I am not paid for the judgment I made," which is based on years of knowledge, experience, and skill.

Many primary-care physicians struggle mightily to keep their practices financially afloat. They are paid much less than specialists. A primary-care doctor in Chicago who sees a patient with diabetes, high blood pressure, and ongoing chest pain is paid $89.64 by Medicare for a thirty-minute visit. A gastroenterologist in Chicago is paid about 253 percent more—$226.63—for a thirty-minute colonoscopy.

If good primary care is not valued, many more people will be caught in the revolving door. Dr. Gardner says, "I would have been perfectly justified to do a CT scan of the chest and abdomen, order more elaborate blood tests, and refer the patient to a surgical specialist to consider a biopsy of the lymph node. No one would have said this was bad medical practice. In fact the standard of practice in my community would have been to do all of this."

Another cost needs to be factored in—the fear factor. Every blood test, CT scan, and biopsy can instill fear while awaiting the day of the test, going through it, and waiting for the results. As one primary-care physician says, "They scare the living daylights out of you for no reason." Dr. Gardner's reassuring approach caused no undue alarm.

Older Americans are especially at risk for receiving medical care that causes them more harm than good because they may have multiple medical conditions. Conscientious primary-care doctors are a bulwark against a treatment tsunami. Dr. Diane Meier of Mount Sinai Hospital in New York, a geriatrician, says that as a primary-care physician she looks at a patient as a whole person, not a collection of isolated organs and individual body parts. Each of the body's systems is interdependent, and a doctor cannot provide good advice to patients without thinking through the interactions of these very complex systems. "Whole person care is not New Age," says Dr. Meier. "It is good medical care."

She remembers a ninety-two-year-old man who fell in his home and fractured his hip and arm. As with many older adults, he had multiple medical conditions. "I got the call from his home health aide and arranged for the man to be seen by an orthopedic surgeon who practiced conservative medicine and did not operate on him, which was the right thing to do. But the patient was put on a nonsteroidal anti-inflammatory drug for pain, which triggered renal failure. The prescribing doctor did not realize that the patient had vascular disease and mild kidney failure—and these drugs reduce blood flow to the kidney. I arrived at the hospital, got the patient off the drugs, and hydrated him. He is now walking."

What would have happened if this ninety-two-year-old man had not had a geriatrician as his doctor? Dr. Meier says, "He would have gone to the ER, been treated by people who did not know him or his medical history, and would very likely have had surgery. The chances of his coming out of it in the same shape he is now—walking—would be low. Everyone taking care of him would have had good intentions, but they would not have seen the big picture. This happens so often that it's routine."

LOOKING ELSEWHERE

Many Americans would like to feel that their doctor is a partner, but they may need to look elsewhere to find people who can help them on their journey to health and well-being. While searching for a solution to a life-threatening medical condition, Jim Gatto from Pennsylvania looked outside the health-care system to find people who could help him. What he found changed his life.

"I thought I was a goner," says Jim, who is retired from Westinghouse. "At age sixty-one, two cardiologists said I would probably need a heart transplant. It scared me to death." Jim had cardiomyopathy, a condition in which the heart muscle becomes enlarged or abnormally thick. As the condition worsens, the heart becomes weaker and less able to supply freshly oxygenated blood to the body. This condition can manifest itself as congestive heart failure, the leading cause of hospitalization among people over the age of sixty-five. About five million people in the United States have congestive heart failure, and about half of them die within five years.

Jim recalls, "I was desperate and needed to do something. The pumping capacity of my heart was only 20 percent. It should be about 55 to 70 percent." If it had been much lower, Jim would have been bedridden or worse.

He went to hear a presentation by Dr. Dean Ornish, a longtime proponent of a healthy lifestyle that embraces a very low-fat diet, physical exercise, stress reduction, and group support. Luckily, during the presentation Jim sat next to a man in his late forties who also had cardiomyopathy and was already changing his lifestyle. The younger man's health had improved dramatically. His experience gave Jim hope that he too could regain his health. "I had been seeing a cardiologist, and when I mentioned I wanted to participate in the Ornish program he had no problem with it," Jim recalls. "But he was not supportive and in fact was completely indifferent. He said, 'Well, go ahead.'"

The program was a big commitment: two days a week, four hours a day. Each day had one hour each of exercise, yoga and meditation, education about food, and group discussion. Because of his history of heart disease, Jim's Blue Cross plan paid the cost of his participation. He stopped eating meat, started yoga and meditation, and began an exercise program. He jokes, "The last time I was in McDonald's was to use the bathroom. I haven't had a hamburger for about twelve years."

The results were dramatic. Jim's heart function improved significantly. Before starting the program he remembers asking his cardiologist whether it would ever improve, and the doctor replied, "Not very likely." Many doctors are dubious about their patients' willingness to do the hard work to change their lifestyle, and people often want a "quick fix." But desperation is a powerful motivator for some people. For Jim, it thrust him on the journey of his life.

About his doctor he says, "He is trained to do procedures such as angioplasty. Many doctors deal with problems rather than prevent them, and I don't think they have time to reflect on how to prevent these things. To prevent the problem, you have to do it on your own."

Keeping good health, and restoring one's health, is a journey. The journey begins with the realization that the human body is not forever. As with any journey, the road will wind its way into territory with unfamiliar languages, customs, and new acquaintances. You may hesitate to stop and ask for help. If you do ask, the directions may be confusing. A person guiding you along the journey may suggest a destination whose road is lined with hucksters of all sorts of gimmicks. Another guide may direct you to a destination where true hospitality and healing await. This is a lifelong journey that never ends. The best journey comes from finding the right people to join you.

PART IV

Every Problem Has a Solution

12 CULL THE OVERUSE, NOT THE PEOPLE

IN HIS ESSAY "The Tragedy of the Commons," Garrett Hardin, a biologist from the University of California at Santa Barbara, wrote: "Picture a pasture open to all. It is to be expected that each herdsman will try to keep as many cattle as possible on the commons. . . . This is the conclusion reached by each and every rational herdsman sharing a commons. Therein is the tragedy. Each man is locked into a system that compels him to increase his herd without limit in a world that is limited. Ruin is the destination toward which all men rush, each pursuing his own best interest."

Many humans graze in the health-care pasture. Hospital CEOs have the incentive to maximize revenue, as do the owners of diagnostic testing facilities, kidney dialysis centers, specialty hospitals, and ambulatory surgical centers.

Doctors who are paid on a piecework basis are motivated to maximize revenue by treating more people and giving more treatment to every patient who walks in the door.

Health-care consultants maximize their revenue when they help hospitals increase the volume of high-cost cardiac, oncology, and orthopedic procedures.

Every pharmaceutical company and medical-device manufacturer has the incentive to maximize sales volume. Oncology companies have every incentive to show oncologists how to maximize their revenue by getting more people into their offices more often.

Patients who have comprehensive health insurance coverage have little incentive to curtail the unnecessary use of medical care.

The White House and members of Congress open the public coffers wider and deeper every year to favor the lobbyists who help them get reelected. Campaign contributions are one of the best bargains in Washington. The return on an investment of thousands of dollars in campaign contributions is millions or billions of dollars of the public's money. Warren Buffett, the Oracle of Omaha and the world's most successful stock market investor, would find it hard to ferret out such a lucrative investment.

Overuse increases the cost of health care for everyone and causes health insurance premiums to skyrocket. Millions of people are denied entry to the health-care pasture because they cannot afford the price to enter. If unnecessary grazing were curtailed, more people could enter the pasture to receive the care they need.

For now, many people are denied entry. A seven-year-old boy diagnosed with leukemia was being treated with chemotherapy. His family had no health insurance, and the hospital required that his parents deposit money into an account at the hospital before their son's treatment could begin. When the money was rapidly depleted, his parents begged family members and neighbors for help. Doctors stopped treatment when the money was gone. His father gently brought his boy home, returning to the hospital sometime later after scraping together meager amounts that were a lifeline for his son.

A sixty-year-old man with lung cancer was uninsured and lacked the money to pay for his treatment. He was self-employed, owned his own business, and was barely making ends meet. To obtain medication for the pain from the cancer, each month he would go to a hospital emergency room at night where he would receive a one month's supply of medicine to help him cope with the pain. One day he bought a gallon of gasoline, poured it around the premises of his small business, and lit a match, setting the building and himself on fire. He died of self-immolation. The hospital had placed a lien on his business for previously unpaid medical expenses. In a final act of defiance, he was determined to prevent the hospital from taking whatever little property he had accumulated during his life.

The seven-year-old boy's name is Dejie, and he was being treated at Beijing Children's Hospital in China. His story was reported in the *Wall Street Journal*. The sixty-year-old small-business owner lived in Minnesota. He received emergency room treatment at a well-known hospital. His story is told by a compassionate physician who first learned of the man's dilemma the day before he died, and had arranged for an ongoing supply of pain medication. When the hospital tried to contact the man the next day to tell him this news, the doctor learned that the man had ended his life.

A primary-care physician on the East Coast says, "I read the article in the *Wall Street Journal*. The same thing that happens in China occurs here in America all the time. They're just more honest about it in China." This doctor had observed a similar circumstance at his hospital. One of his patients was being treated for cancer by an oncologist. After losing her private insurance coverage, her oncologist refused to continue treatment. To abandon a patient is one of the worst things a physician can do. The woman's primary-care physician says, "It's not as if the oncologist was going broke. It's about sending your kids to summer camp, or deciding between a new or used BMW." The young woman was eligible for health insurance coverage through a public program and was treated at a hospital clinic. She eventually succumbed to the disease.

The *Wall Street Journal* reported Dejie's story in an article about medical treatment in China, which highlighted a Chinese cabinet-level think-tank analysis of the challenges facing the country's health-care system. The government report acknowledges the inequities between rich and poor and the consequences of a Darwinian health-care system where everyone must fend for themselves in a cash-for-treatment system.

Growing numbers of Americans who have no insurance or are underinsured are also fending for themselves in the U.S. cash-for-treatment system. Excluded from the pasture, they embark on a search that takes them to places they never imagined.

The mountains of Taos, New Mexico, remind Carlo Gislimberti of his hometown in the Dolomite Mountains in northern Italy. "The moment I saw the mountains, I knew this is where I was meant to be," he says. He and his wife, Siobhan, set down roots in Taos years ago. An accomplished chef, Carlo established a four-star restaurant that blended his native old world Italian cooking with a southwestern flair.

"In April 2005, while doing landscaping around the restaurant, I was having difficulty breathing," he says. "I am 'old news' in the heart department." Carlo had a history of heart problems, including two heart attacks, and at age forty-eight he had triple-vessel coronary angioplasty to open clogged arteries. With the new bout of breathing difficulty, he went to a cardiologist and learned that "I could drop dead any moment." He required immediate bypass surgery.

Carlo had lost his health insurance coverage several years earlier, after the angioplasty procedure. He could have purchased other health insurance, but the premium was $2,000 a month. Carlo says he had to make a choice between paying himself a salary that would support his wife and himself or going uninsured. He chose to take the risk of no insurance.

The bypass surgery would cost $150,000, a stunning amount of money. Carlo would have to sell his restaurant, which was his livelihood and his home, as he and his wife lived upstairs. "I was facing financial death or death by heart attack," he says.

His wife searched the internet for a cardiology center to find a place where Carlo might have the surgery at a reasonable cost. She finally found a hospital in New Delhi, India. The cardiac surgeon there had received his medical training in New York, which gave her confidence, and she made arrangements for her husband to have surgery in New Delhi.

"I've trekked in Nepal three times and knew what to expect in a country such as India," Carlo says. "It's a totally different world, and you have to be prepared." He and

Siobhan arrived in New Delhi and were taken immediately to the hospital. Once they stepped inside, "it was like a hospital in Houston or New York," he says. "The amenities were unbelievable. The staff was excellent, the food was excellent. A barber came every day. We brought a laptop with us so we could communicate with everyone back home, and they even helped us connect it."

After days of tests, Carlo remembers how "the psychological shield I had built to prepare myself in case something happened chipped away every day." His condition was worse than expected. He was in surgery for seven hours and had triple-bypass surgery. The cost of the surgery and twenty days in the hospital was $10,000. He had paid the hospital $15,000 in advance and was reimbursed $5,000.

Carlo and his wife returned home a month after the surgery. His health would not permit him to continue a chef's grueling schedule. With life at a crossroads, he embarked with fervor on what he calls the "Third Age." His relentless creativity is now expressed as an artist in brilliant landscapes of the Sangre de Cristo Mountains of New Mexico, the Himalayan mountains of Nepal, and the shores of California.

When asked what he thinks of traveling thousands of miles away from home to a poor country to obtain affordable health care, Carlo says, "It's a disgrace. I love this country. I have been able to make a good life here. But when it comes to health, human beings shouldn't be treated differently, no matter who they are."

The American health-care system has plenty of money to take care of Carlo and the millions of other people who need medical care. Millions of dollars were spent on unnecessary procedures performed on Ron Spurgeon's heart and the hearts of hundreds of people in Redding, California, jeopardizing their life and their health. Meanwhile the system does not pay for surgery for people like Carlo who really need it.

The number of Americans now traveling overseas for essential medical care is just a trickle. How much this so-called medical tourism grows will depend on the number of people who are desperate for medical care and have some means to pay for it. If cost trends continue, and as employers continue to cut back on health insurance coverage for employees, more Americans will have no choice but to find their own way in an increasingly Darwinian health-care system.

Medical tourism is not a picnic, as its name might imply. Images may spring to mind of recovering patients sitting under palm trees and sipping mango juice, yet they belie the reality that medical treatment is always a serious matter. For Carlo, it was a matter of life and death.

GOING TO THE HOSPITAL? PACK YOUR PASSPORT

One of the people who are bullish on Americans going global for their health care is Tom Keesling, president and co-founder of IndUShealth, a Raleigh, North Carolina–based enterprise that promotes medical tourism. A former hospital CEO in the United States, Keesling says that fifteen million Americans with incomes of more than $75,000 have no health insurance, and they are his target market. The IndUShealth website lists the costs of common surgical procedures such as knee-replacement surgery, which it says has a median cost of $45,000 and can be done in a state-of-the-art hospital in India for $8,000 to $13,000, including travel. Greater savings can be realized on high-cost procedures such as a heart-valve replacement, which is listed at $125,000 in the United States and can be had for less than $15,000, travel included.

More hospitals overseas are becoming accredited by Joint Commission International (JCI), a Chicago-based subsidiary of the Joint Commission, the organization that accredits U.S. hospitals. Karen Timmons, president and chief executive officer of JCI, observes that "As leading hospitals overseas become accredited, more hospitals are interested in accreditation. We are working now in eighty countries and have opened offices in Geneva, Dubai, and Singapore."

Even people with good health insurance may not be immune from having to travel thousands of miles from home. Health insurance company executives are visiting hospitals in India, Singapore, and Thailand to survey the prospects for sending Americans overseas for medical care at a discount. In South Carolina, Blue Cross and Blue Shield is one of the first insurers to launch a subsidiary, Companion Global Healthcare, to do just that. The company will schedule appointments, make travel arrangements, and answer questions about services and prices for overseas medical care.

Keesling believes it will not be long before private insurers offer discounts to people who choose to go global. His business is betting on it. His excitement grows when he describes Boeing's new 787 Dreamliner that will carry three hundred passengers aloft for long-distance air travel. In the brave new world of health care, the seats may be filled with people going to the hospital, not the Taj Mahal.

Keesling says, "I've talked to so many people in health care who are banging their heads against the wall, not knowing what to do. There are too many vested interests, and you can't cut through them. The only way to fix the system is to have a lot of pain, and politically, no one wants to do that. So let's try something different where we can get high-quality care at an affordable price. It's one of those disruptive innovations."

Will going global successfully challenge mainstream U.S. health care to become efficient? Or is it a cheaper alternative for people who are kept out of the pasture? Going global is not a challenge to American hospitals, as many of them would probably prefer that uninsured and underinsured people not show up on their doorstep.

How many more people in America are like Carlo and the man who set himself on fire? The U.S. government does not count the number of people who need lifesaving medical care but cannot afford it.

As a growing number of middle-class Americans are being locked out of affordable medical care, people higher up the food chain will soon be joining them. It is a club that no one wants to join. Higher-income workers who think they are untouchable may need to think again. Jobs for architects, accountants, and other professions that have been stepping-stones to a comfortable life for many Americans are vulnerable, as the economic downturn has demonstrated. As good jobs go, so goes health insurance. Whatever health insurance coverage Americans have will continue to shrink and may become a shadow of its former self.

MEDICAL REFUGEES

Imagine having a heart that needs repair, but the only hospital willing to perform an affordable surgery is a twenty-hour plane ride away from family, friends, and familiar surroundings. Imagine driving to an airport with bags and passport packed and passing by state-of-the-art hospitals where cardiac surgery is performed by doctors who are the best in the world. Imagine knowing that gaining access to the gleaming steel towers and light-filled atriums of these hospitals is impossible because the entry fees are too high.

Imagine realizing that after years of working hard and paying taxes, a portion of those taxes may have been used to subsidize the training of the doctors inside the steel towers, perhaps the construction of the building itself, or the cost of the heart surgeries that are being performed at that very moment.

Imagine reading on the way to the airport the *Harvard Business Review*'s article, "Why U.S. Health Care Costs Aren't Too High," which debunks the notion that affordable health care in the United States is a problem. According to this purported breakthrough idea, "At least for the foreseeable future, health care in the United States is an economic, a societal and an affordable good." Imagine writing a letter to the editor of the *Harvard Business Review* upon returning home to explain the reality of the other health-care America. For now, though, none of this matters on the road to the airport to repair a broken heart.

For generations, America has been a refuge to millions throughout the world seeking to escape religious and political persecution, poverty, and starvation. Now, in an unprecedented shift, Americans are learning that their mother country is no longer a refuge. They leave the United States not for political reasons but because they are sick and may die, and need affordable health care that is not accessible to them. It is an act of desperation. Organizations promoting medical tourism are helping them leave. They are not charities, and neither are the hospitals springing up overseas waiting for America's sick and tired to have their hearts healed. They are profit-making enterprises.

On the Statue of Liberty, the words of Emma Lazarus's poem "The New Colossus" are inscribed. "Give me your tired, your poor, your huddled masses . . ." America no longer wants its health-care poor. It is shipping them elsewhere. They are health-care refugees. This is where we are headed in health-care America. But the United States has a choice. We can cull the people, or we can cull overuse.

13 THE OTHER INCONVENIENT TRUTH

THE DOCUMENTARY FILM *An Inconvenient Truth* vividly paints a frightening picture of planet Earth changing in dramatic ways as a consequence of human activity. One need not be a scientist to recognize the shifts in the Earth's climate. Melting Arctic glaciers menace the homes of native Alaskans while tornadoes whip through Brooklyn, New York. Scientists predict hundred-year floods every ten years in New York City, drowning the subway system. Americans no longer need fear a "Silent Spring," the startling image that Rachel Carson gave the world in her 1962 book about pesticides. Now the fear is that there will be no spring as we have known it.

The creators of *An Inconvenient Truth* say that the turning point in the global warming debate occurred with the realization that the world can no longer afford to see the topic as a political issue. Global warming, they say, has become the greatest moral challenge facing world civilization. This shift from a political to a moral issue creates the will for people to change. It gives a moral purpose to the work that lies ahead.

What does global warming have to do with health care? At first glance, not much. A closer look reveals that both health and the environment are compelling issues of our time that affect the survival of life itself. People become unglued when threats to life are in our midst. When the threats become morally unacceptable in hearts and minds, a collective voice begins to emerge that challenges the status quo.

What would a documentary of "The Other Inconvenient Truth" reveal? It would show home video of Michael Skolnik, a six-foot-four-inch "infant in diapers" being lovingly cared for day and night by his mother and father in the aftermath of needless brain surgery. He died almost three years later.

It would show Mary Anne, the scientist from Massachusetts, who lives with a body she wishes "had gone to the morgue" the day she had an unnecessary and botched hysterectomy.

It would show the scar on Ron's chest, which is like that of a gutted trout.

Our country will not be successful in curbing the vast misallocation of health-care resources if reform is viewed as a political and financial issue. The political battles will be the same. Members of Congress will continue to be held hostage by industry lobbyists demanding Medicare reimbursement for a newfangled diagnostic test or device that is not an improvement over a cheaper, existing alternative. The hostages will be freed and will be reelected when they relent and agree to have Medicare pay for it. The ransom money, or peace-buying, will continue to be paid by the little people, the taxpayers, the bighearted backbone of the country. As Dr. Donald Berwick has written, we "buy ourselves peace through the allocation of waste."

THE NONSOLUTION

The health-care industry and financial services companies like to say that patients should act more like consumers and bear a greater share of the cost of their health care. By becoming more cost conscious, proponents believe, consumers will make more informed decisions and spend more frugally. This is how the industry proposes to check the growth of the green monster.

As more people pay directly with their own money, however, they will have an impact only on the margins of health-care spending. The green monster is too big and too voracious to be curbed by an individual consumer. Putting more of the financial burden for health care on consumers is a solution that is little different from trying to control Pentagon spending by requiring soldiers to pay for their own body armor. The soldiers' spending from their own pockets will have no effect on the billions of dollars spent on big-ticket items. These spending decisions are made higher up in the hierarchies of American government and in the companies that sell to them.

When consumers become patients, they come to depend on doctors and nurses. The word "patient" comes from the Latin word *patior*, "to suffer." Suffering from the burden of disease, especially one that sparks fear of mortality, can impede our ability to act in our own best interests. In the midst of suffering, we trust and believe because we are scared to death.

When hundreds of Californians in Redding were told they required heart bypass surgery and other heart procedures, they believed they needed them and might die without them. When Helen Haskell of South Carolina asked questions about an elective surgery for her son, she believed what doctors told her. When Mr. Goode was told that knee-replacement surgery would enable him to go fishing, he believed it. When Patty Skolnik was told her that son, Michael, needed brain surgery, she believed the doctor.

Health care can never be a market like any other market because doctors, nurses, and others have knowledge and experience that patients and their families can never have. The green monster stands by, licking its chops. A physician has said about patients, "They are like lambs to slaughter."

Financial services companies are pumping more fuel into the medical arms race. Patients in some states can now go to their doctor's office or hospital to apply for a health-care credit card. Citibank's Citi Health Card is marketed to doctors who are encouraged to have their patients apply. According to Citibank's Citi Health Card website, the benefits to doctors are financially advantageous. "For patients, the biggest obstacle to getting treatments is often financial concerns," Citibank tells doctors. "Now you can improve sales . . . [and] increase the number of procedures scheduled. . . . With flexible monthly payments, patients have the opportunity to start treatments they might otherwise delay and enable them to choose more comprehensive treatments because they can spread payments over time." Citibank tells doctors that when their patients apply for the credit card, "We'll provide a fast decision . . . so treatment can begin immediately."

One can imagine a doctor telling a patient that he or she has cancer, then handing over a credit card application so that the chemotherapy costs may be charged. Americans are already maxed out on credit cards, so it's hard to see how a credit card that is advertised as having a 26.9 percent interest rate is a viable solution for families looking to pay for medical expenses. Meanwhile the patient with cancer is in no position to negotiate or shop for lower-priced treatment when his or her life is at stake. This matters little to financial services companies. The temptation to obtain a small sliver of total health-care spending is irresistible.

A GREAT WALL OF DEBT

If no action is taken to curb overuse, the country will be surrounded by an even higher "great wall of debt" as the federal government borrows from China and other countries to help pay today's health-care bills and other expenses. A portion of American workers' paychecks is being sent to China and other countries to pay the interest on the debt our government now owes.

It might be defensible for the U.S. government to borrow money if it were used for medical care that yielded real value, such as cataract surgery that allows the blind to see, orthopedic surgery that permits the lame to walk, and heart surgery to fix a broken heart so it can continue its beat. Instead, too much borrowed money is being used to pay for the poking and prodding of the human body that yields no benefit and increases the possibility of harm.

If the country spends 25 percent of the nation's income on health care in the year 2025—and that's the amount we are on track to spend—there will be no money for all the other things that Americans have come to expect from their government. The country will drown in its own debt, sink in its economic standing in the world, and resemble a third-world debtor nation. The green monster will be triumphant as it quietly yet deftly drags the country under the rising water from the melting fiscal glaciers.

Health policy experts are working diligently to find technical solutions to reform the "do something" culture. Many others are working overtime to bring health care into the twenty-first century with electronic health records. These improvements are essential but not sufficient, because they don't address the root cause.

Garrett Hardin writes, "An implicit and almost universal assumption of discussions published in professional and semi-popular scientific journals is that the problem under discussion has a technical solution. A technical solution may be defined as one that requires a change only in the techniques of the natural sciences, demanding little or nothing in the way of change in human values of ideas of morality."

RECLAIMING THE MORAL PURPOSE

To live a long and healthy life is an aspiration of the human spirit that transcends generations, cultures, languages, and political party affiliation. The holy books of the major religions of the world speak of this aspiration, as do poets and our own human hearts. Nations establish health-care systems to allow their citizens to fulfill a universal desire for life, freedom from the bondage of illness, and the pursuit of happiness. Can the moral purpose be reclaimed?

Many compassionate physicians, nurses, and health-care leaders dedicate their lives to the noble work of healing the sick. When the health-care system works well, millions of Americans are restored to health. As one physician has said, "It's the closest thing to God's work." Americans on both sides of the bedrails—conscientious professionals and the public—are starving for a moral compass in health care. How noble it would be to feed the people, not the green monster.

14   A TEN-STEP RECOVERY PLAN

HERE ARE TEN STEPS to halt the overuse of medical care. The health of our nation's economy, and our own pocketbooks, depends on it. In fact it's hard to think of anything more sensible than to stop spending money on things that can cause more harm than good—or no good at all.

1. SHINE A LIGHT ON THE OUTLIERS

Medicare should regularly and publicly report the top ten communities in the United States that show three and four times the national average of major surgical procedures and diagnostic testing. By shining a light on the outliers, they will no longer remain in the shadows. Organizations like Consumers Union can explain this information to the public so they can avoid being caught in the trap of overuse. If Ron Spurgeon, the California millwright, had known that his community's rate of heart bypass surgery was the highest in the country, he might have pulled the emergency brake and obtained a second or third opinion before consenting to bypass surgery for his nonexistent heart disease.

2. AUDIT THE OUTLIERS

Any hospital that performs a medical procedure at a rate triple or quadruple the national average should automatically trigger Medicare to conduct an independent review to determine if patients are benefiting. Exceptions may be made for hospitals that are centers of excellence whose patients come from throughout the country for treatment. The results of these reviews should be made public and easily accessible to members of the pertinent community. When Redding Hospital in California was performing heart procedures at a rate far higher than the national average, no one intervened, even though Medicare had information that showed sky-high heart bypass surgery rates. To rely on a patient to pull the emergency brake, which happened in this case, is not a solution. A systematic, pro-active approach is needed to pull the plug on overuse.

3. SET A NATIONAL GOAL TO REDUCE INAPPROPRIATE DIAGNOSTIC IMAGING TESTS

The American public is exposed to unprecedented amounts of radiation from diagnostic imaging tests. The American College of Radiology has reported that the annual collective dose of radiation from medical diagnostic tests in the United States is estimated to be roughly equivalent to the total worldwide collective dose generated by the nuclear catastrophe at Chernobyl. The group presumes that this exposure will lead to an increased incidence of cancer. Meanwhile, experts estimate that one-third of the imaging tests performed on adults are unnecessary, and more than one million children have unnecessary tests. The secretary of Health and Human Services should establish a goal and time period for reducing unnecessary diagnostic imaging tests for which Medicare pays.

4. STOP PAYING FOR THINGS THAT DON'T WORK

Medicare should pay for surgeries and other procedures only if evidence exists that people benefit. Most Americans probably think that Medicare does this already. It does not. Medicare did a smart thing when it helped fund a study to learn if patients with emphysema benefited from a surgery called lung-volume reduction. Some people lived longer but others did not, including 8 percent who died, a very high mortality rate. Medicare established a policy that it would pay for the surgery only when it was performed on people who would benefit. This is smart public policy that should be adopted broadly.

5. FIND OUT WHAT WORKS

A rarely spoken truth in twenty-first-century health care in the most advanced country in the world is that too often doctors do not know whether the care they provide to their patients does them any good. When physicians systematically examine the care they provide to their patients and share that information with colleagues and the public, they can learn what works, and so will we. "This is the best way to find out if we as doctors are providing the best care to patients," says Dr. Paul Miles, vice president for quality improvement at the American Board of Pediatrics. Enormous progress has been made in the treatment of cancer in children because doctors have shared this kind of information. It is a model for learning what works and what does not. Dr. Miles says, "For two thousand years we have said, 'Trust me, I'm a doctor.' We can no longer say that. We need to be willing to show our data on patient outcomes to the public. They are saying, 'Doc, I do trust you, but show me the data.'" He's right.

6. SPEND MONEY FOR PUBLIC INFORMATION ABOUT TREATMENT OPTIONS

Public investments should be made in developing evidence-based information to help people make treatment choices that are right for them. The DVDs and other materials developed by the Foundation for Informed Medical Decision Making are a model for the type of information to which every consumer should have access. The videos can be made available on the National Library of Medicine website. Currently the website contains videos of surgeries being performed on real patients. A great service would be to provide the public with information to weigh the risks and benefits of surgery and other treatment options. The videos can also be made available through online DVD rental services such as Netflix, which would make them easily accessible to the public.

7. GIVE HEALTH INSURANCE DISCOUNTS TO INFORMED PATIENTS

Medicare and health insurance companies should consider discounts to people who face a decision about medical treatment and who become informed about their options and the risks and benefits. Studies have shown that when people are informed, they make better decisions that are right for them, and they often choose less invasive and less costly interventions. Organizations such as AARP have on-line driver safety courses that can be taken in the comfort of one's own home. Similarly, people who are deciding about a treatment or test should be able to access online information about treatment options provided by an independent organization that has no financial stake in the treatment decision. Upon completion, health insurance companies can offer informed patients a discount on their premium or waive deductibles.

8. RATE HOSPITALS ON HOW WELL THEY EXPLAIN TREATMENT OPTIONS

Hospitals should be rated for how well they explain treatment options to patients. When *Consumer Reports* rates a product as poor it receives a black dot, and when a product is rated excellent it receives a red dot, so that consumers can easily understand performance outcomes. Hospitals should get a black dot if they do not explain to patients their options and their risks and benefits in an understandable fashion.

9. ASK: "WHAT ARE THE TOP TEN THINGS WE SHOULD STOP DOING?"

Imagine if doctors, nurses, hospital CEOs, and the millions of other people who work in hospitals, physicians' offices, medical device companies, and other health-care organizations were asked, "What are the top ten tests, treatments, and procedures that we should stop doing because they cause more harm than good?" They could submit their ideas on the website of a public-spirited organization and rank them in importance for stopping overuse. The response would likely be huge, because many conscientious health-care workers see unnecessary treatment every day but feel powerless to stop it.

Also, imagine if people who have had unnecessary treatment could share their personal stories of overuse and any harm that occurred. Doctors and nurses who have observed overuse could share their experiences too. Imagine if these stories were compared side-by-side with those of people who need medical treatment but cannot afford it. The comparison would make us see how crazy the current system is. Who knows, we might be motivated to stop the excess and recycle it for good use.

10. STOP FEE-FOR-SERVICE PAYMENT FOR MEDICAL CARE

Medicare and private insurers' methods of payment to doctors, hospitals, and other health-care providers must change. Paying them for each individual unit of service invites overuse and corruption. Opposition to reform will naturally be deafening. Lionhearted courage will be required to establish a payment system that rewards care that measurably improves people's lives and their quality of life at an affordable cost. If we don't change, our country and our families will financially bleed to death.

In his essay "Tragedy of the Commons," Garrett Hardin wrote that by recognizing resources as a commons that requires management, "we can preserve and nurture other more previous freedoms." Our excessively rich health-care system exists at the expense of two precious freedoms: the economic and financial sustainability of our country and our families, and the pursuit of a good life with the blessings of health and good health care. We all have these aspirations, including those who are wealthy but who could someday be poorer from too much waste. If we choose, we can reclaim these precious freedoms so that all may prosper in the years ahead.

15 TWENTY SMART WAYS TO PROTECT YOURSELF

A WISE PERSON once said, "There are three kinds of people in the world: those who will do you good, those who will do you harm, and those who will do you neither good nor harm." The same is true with health care. It can do much good. It can also do harm, or neither harm nor good.

Today's health care is not your grandmother's health care. The good news is that you can now be empowered with more information than ever before about staying healthy and receiving the care you need. But now, the business of health care intertwines money and medicine, and it can be hard to know whether what you are getting is good medicine or just good for business. The stakes have never been higher for you to make yourself an educated health-care consumer. Research shows that when people are fully informed of their options and the risks and benefits, they choose care that is medically appropriate but less invasive and intensive than what their doctor has recommended.

This is especially good news because it means that you can be in the driver's seat and receive the care that is right for you, no more and no less.

If you think you can't make a difference and the challenge is just too daunting, think again. Maybe you never got an "A" in high school biology, but you *are* an expert in what is important to *you*. Here are practical suggestions to guide you on your journey to health.

1. REMEMBER THE DONUT SHOP

Remember the story of the young chief operating officer who said to a doctor in his hospital, "We are like a donut shop. Our job is to sell donuts. If we don't sell a lot of donuts, we go out of business. Your job . . . is to convince patients they need to be in the hospital. . . ." Many altruistic people go to work every day to provide the best care they can. But many organizations where they work are motivated by one aim: maximize revenue. You, the patient, are the source of that revenue. Realize that health care is a moneymaking business. In the coming years, many providers of medical care will capitalize on the growing number of people who are getting older and a system that financially rewards overuse. Your expectations about eternal youth will fuel the use of more medical care. For many Americans, this perfect storm will cause more harm than good. Don't get caught in the storm.

2. DON'T BE A CASH COW

If you have comprehensive health insurance, you could be at greater risk for needless medical treatment because you have the means to pay for it. Health insurance has given people access to health care. But now health insurance is a way for providers to gain access to patients. Hospitals and other health-care providers want patients who have good insurance that covers high-cost procedures. So if you have insurance, be aware that some providers of medical care may see your health insurance card as a credit card they can use to benefit their bottom line.

3. WATCH OUT FOR THE WALLET BIOPSY

A wallet biopsy is a procedure that might be performed without your consent. It happens when hospitals and doctors assess how much treatment your insurance will cover. Many good doctors will want to consider your financial situation in helping you get the best care you can afford. Others may see your wallet as an opportunity.

4. THE BIOPSY YOU DO WANT

Never allow a doctor to tell you that you have cancer if a biopsy has not been performed that confirms the presence of disease. Tom Vallier, whose doctor told him he had cancer and performed surgery without confirming the diagnosis with a biopsy, says that it's not enough to trust a doctor who says you have cancer and doesn't confirm it with a biopsy. Tom's wife, Deandra, says, "Trust but verify." That's good advice.

5. DON'T LET THEM MARINATE YOUR MIND: BE MEDIA SAVVY

You need to be media savvy and know how to distinguish marketing glitz from accurate information that might benefit you and your family. The best independent analysis of health-care news is HealthNewsReview.org. Based at the University of Minnesota, it reviews news stories that make a therapeutic claim about treatments, procedures, new drugs or devices, diagnostic and screening tests, and vitamins and nutritional supplements. News stories are graded and critiques are published on its website. You will find balanced critiques of health stories reported on television programs such as *Today* and *Good Morning America*, and in newspapers and magazines such as the *New York Times* and *Time*.

6. FIND OUT IF YOU ARE GETTING SCIENCE OR GUESSWORK

One of the best questions you can ask a doctor who recommends a treatment, test, or procedure is, "How do you know it will work for me?" If the reply you receive is something like, "Oh, I've done this procedure many times," or "So many of my patients do well," that's not good enough. You should expect a more complete answer. Your physician should explain the procedure, treatment options (including those that he or she does *not* perform), the evidence about what works and what doesn't, and their risks and benefits. If you have a conversation like this with your doctor, you will have valuable information to help you make a decision that is right for you.

7. DON'T SUCCUMB TO HIGH-PRESSURE TACTICS

If a treatment recommended to you is optional and not an emergency, don't give in to pressure to make a decision immediately. Questioning the advice of a doctor can be difficult, especially when you are dealing with a painful condition, illness, and uncertainty. A good doctor will not pressure you to do something you are not sure about. He or she will help you make a decision that is right for you.

8. ASK YOURSELF THE MILLION-DOLLAR QUESTION

At some point in your life you may face a decision that is very difficult to make, and you won't know what to do. You may feel bombarded by options and opinions. Whatever the circumstance, ask yourself, "What is important to me in my life right now?" As you answer this question, think about your life, how you live your life, and the values that guide you. Listen to the voice inside and follow your gut instinct. You are not an expert about medical care, but you are an expert about you. A good doctor will listen to what is important to you and help you make a decision that feels right.

9. GET CONNECTED: LEARN WHAT DOCTORS DON'T TELL YOU

Go online and find a reputable online community of people like you who are living with the same condition or have made a decision that you must make. Knowing that you are not alone can calm your fears. You will learn how others live with their condition or treatment and where they have found help. You can forge your own path to receive the care you need and avoid the treatment you don't.

10. IT'S ALL ABOUT THE NETWORK

Searching for a health-care provider that is right for you can be like looking for a job. Networking with family, friends, co-workers, and neighbors can help you find the place and the people who are right for you. Experienced nurses can be a good source of information when you want to find a good doctor. Ask them about the doctor or hospital they would use if they were in your situation. Nurses talk among themselves, and they are patients too.

11. APPOINT A COORDINATOR-IN-CHIEF

In twenty-first-century health care, there is no mother in the system. You will need to be the coordinator-in-chief of your care or appoint someone who can connect the dots among doctors, lab reports, and treatments. Even if you have doctors who are competent and caring, you need to fill in the cracks in the system so you do not fall into them. Doctors can give you advice, but you need to put all the pieces together. Also, you need to question the work of the many moving parts in the system, because it is rare to find a person who will do that for you. The task is daunting. Most of us would rather shut our eyes and hope that someone will take care of us. In today's health-care marketplace, it helps to be realistic. Your life may depend on it.

12. HOW TO LEARN ABOUT YOUR TREATMENT OPTIONS

The Foundation for Informed Medical Decision Making is one of the best sources of information about treatment options and their risks and benefits. Its approach is "just the facts," and it has no bias or vested interest other than helping people make a decision they believe is right for them.

The foundation creates DVDs and other information on topics such as how to choose the right treatment for herniated disks, heart disease, and breast cancer, and whether men should have the PSA test for prostate cancer. You may be able to obtain the videos from your health plan or doctor. If not, contact the foundation directly about obtaining a copy to review in return for completing a questionnaire about the video.

13. KNOW THAT THE TREATMENT YOU GET MAY DEPEND ON WHERE YOU LIVE

Find out if your community has high rates of different types of surgery. Go to the website of the *Dartmouth Atlas*, which shows the large differences in how often common medical procedures—such as knee replacement, heart bypass, angioplasty, and back surgery—are performed. If your back hurts, for example, and your doctor recommends back surgery, check to see if your community is listed and if it has a high rate of this kind of surgery. If you live in Mason City, Iowa, or Bend, Oregon, you will notice that these communities have higher rates of back surgery than San Francisco and Honolulu. This information will not help you make a medical decision that is right for you, but it will make you aware that the treatment your doctor recommends may depend not on you and your medical condition but on how doctors in your community practice medicine.

14. FIND OUT WHAT DOCTORS SAY ABOUT *YOU*

When you have a doctor's appointment, ask for a copy of your medical record and read it. You will find out if your record reflects your understanding of your condition and treatment. Conscientious doctors give their patients a copy. Your medical record may be incomplete or contain errors, and you can try to correct them. At least you will know what doctors are saying about you.

15. KEEP TRACK OF YOUR X-RAYS, CT SCANS, AND OTHER DIAGNOSTIC IMAGING TESTS

One of six adults reports that his or her doctor ordered a medical test such as an x-ray that had already been done. Because the National Institutes of Health has designated x-rays a carcinogen, keep track of the x-rays as well as CT scans and nuclear medicine tests you have had. Go to the American Nuclear Society web site, www.ans.org, which has a radiation dose chart, to learn about the amount of radiation exposure from common diagnostic imaging tests.

16. WHAT TO DO IF YOU SUSPECT FINANCIAL CONFLICTS OF INTEREST

Financial conflicts of interest are pervasive in health care. Doctors who recommend tests or procedures may have a financial stake in the MRI facility, lab, surgery center, or hospital. Ethical guidelines from the American Medical Association require them to disclose financial conflicts of interest to their patients, but it rarely happens. Trisha Torrey, a former teacher and now a patient advocate, fended off unwanted chemotherapy for a nonexistent cancer. Her advice is, "If a doctor has a financial stake in the treatment he or she recommends, always obtain a second opinion. Most doctors will say that their financial interest does not affect their judgment. Most patients would say it *can* affect their judgment. So get another opinion."

17. GIVE BACK

If you are an overachiever, share your knowledge and wisdom. You can make a difference in someone's life. You can do this in online forums such as the Association of Cancer Online Resources (ACOR) and other reputable online communities of people who help one another every day. Your experience of grappling with a disease or medical condition may help someone else cope with daily challenges. You will benefit too, because helping others is always good medicine.

If you are a super overachiever, join the consumer network of the Cochrane Collaboration, a global network of volunteers who are experts in their field. They review the strongest research available about health-care interventions and can help patients and health-care professionals make informed decisions. Their reviews are the gold standard and are published online. Any active consumer can join the Cochrane Consumer Network to help ensure that medical care is based on the best evidence. To learn more, go to http://www.cochrane.org/consumers/about.htm.

18. LESS MAY BE MORE THAN YOU EVER IMAGINED

Prevention is one of the best defenses against unnecessary medical care. When Ralph Nill of Pittsburgh learned at age fifty-eight that he needed a heart transplant, he was scared and desperate. He changed his diet, became more physically active, and learned how to reduce stress. He became part of a community of people who were trying to change their lifestyle, and they supported and motivated him. Ralph no longer has chest pain, and his cardiologist said he no longer needs a new heart. Now, at age seventy, his advice to his children and others is, "You have the advantage of knowing you can prevent major heart damage by changing your diet and lifestyle while you are still young. I would give anything to go back and do it differently. I can't do that, but you can." And yes, you can.

19. THINK HEALTH

National Geographic reporters trotted around the globe to find people who have lived the longest and to ferret out their secrets of a long life. In the mountain villages of Sardinia, Italy, the islands of Okinawa, and among Seventh-Day Adventists in Loma Linda, California, they found people with exceptional longevity. Reaching the age of one hundred is not out of the ordinary in these communities, and the years of life are healthy as people suffer only a fraction of the diseases that commonly cut lives short elsewhere. Their health and longevity is explained by close ties to family and friends and a reason to wake up in the morning—things money can't buy.

20. ABIDE BY THE WISDOM OF THE AGES

Around 500 B.C., Gautama Siddhartha lived in India. Today he is known as Buddha. In words handed down through the centuries, he said, "Do not believe in anything simply because you have heard it. Do not believe in anything simply because it is spoken and rumored by many. Do not believe in traditions because they have been handed down for many generations. But after observation and analysis, when you find that anything agrees with reason and is conducive to the good and benefit of one and all, then accept it and live up to it."

Notes

Introduction

17 "one-third of Americans say": Sabrina K. H. How, Anthony Shih, Jennifer Lau, and Cathy Schoen, "Public View on U.S. Health System Organization: A Call for New Directions," Data Brief, August 2008, 4. The Commonwealth Fund, http://www.commonwealthfund.org/usr_doc/Public_Views_SurveyPg_8-4-08.pdf?section=4056. Accessed August 31, 2008.

25 "From the ability to not let well enough alone": Robert Hutchison, letter to the editor, *British Medical Journal*, March 21, 1953, 671.

1: Voices in the Wilderness

30 "For half a century": John Wennberg, "Physician Uncertainty, Specialty Ideology, and Second Opinion Prior to Tonsillectomy," *Pediatrics*, vol 59, no 6, June 1977, 952. http://pediatrics.aappublications.org/cgi/content/abstract/59/6/952. Accessed April 11, 2009.

30 "In 1976": U.S. Congress, House Subcommittee on Oversight and Investigations, "Cost and Quality of Health Care: Unnecessary Surgery," Washington, D.C.: U.S. Government Printing Office, 1976.

30 "Seventeen percent of endoscopies were performed": M. R. Chassin, et al., "Does Inappropriate Use Explain Geographic Variations in the Use of Health Care Services? A Study of Three

Procedures," *Journal of the American Medical Association*, vol 258, no 18, November 13, 1987. http://jama.ama-assn.org/cgi/content/abstract/258/18/2533. Accessed August 31, 2008.

31 "A *Wall Street Journal*": "The Case Against Stents: New Studies Hint at Overuse," *Wall Street Journal*, January 23, 2007, 1. http://online.wsj.com/article/SB116952187425084569.html. Accessed May 25, 2008.

31 "The *New York Times* reported": Reed Abelson, "Heart Procedure Is Off the Charts in an Ohio City," *New York Times*, August 18, 2006. http://www.nytimes.com/2006/08/18/business/18stent.html. Accessed August 31, 2008.

31 "Brody wrote": Jane Brody, "A Fight for Full Disclosure of the Possible Pain," *New York Times*, March 8, 2005, F7.

31 "In Hilton Head, South Carolina": Peter Frost, "Suit Alleges Medicare Defrauded," *Hilton Head Island Packet*, October 9, 2006. See also Peter Frost, "Prosecutors Can't Find Ex-cardiologist Accused of Fraud," *Hilton Head Island Packet*, November 23, 2006.

32 "The *Miami Herald* reported": John Dorschner, "Neurosurgeon, Hospital Settle Whistle-blower Case," *Miami Herald*, July 27, 2007.

32 "The *Minot* (North Dakota) *Daily News*": Dave Caldwell, "Bottineau Woman Files Malpractice Suit Against Trinity," *Minot Daily News*, March 9, 2007. http://www.minotdailynews.com/news/articles.asp?articleID=9481. Accessed March 14, 2007.

32 "The newspaper alleged": Gabe Semenza, "Are Doctors' Morals for Sale?" *Victoria Advocate*, March 11, 2007.

32 "Debra Ness, president": Debra Ness, president, National Partnership for Women and Families, U.S. Senate Health, Education, Labor and Pensions Committee, January 10, 2007.

2: A Doctor's Tale

39 "Nearly 80 percent": David O. Weber, "Unethical Business Practices in U.S. Health Care Alarm Physician Leaders," *Physician Executive*, March–April 2005, 8.

39 "When asked whether their colleagues": Weber, "Unethical Business Practices," 8.

40 "Our community has the highest rate": Bill Steiger, "Doctors Say Many Obstacles Block Paths to Patient Safety," *Physician Executive*, May–June 2007, 10.

3: How Did We Come to This?

42 "The National Center for Health Statistics": *2006 National Hospital Discharge Survey*, U.S. Department of Health and Human Services, Centers for Disease Control and Prevention, National Center for Health Statistics, no 5, July 30, 2008, 16.

42 "More than 120": Sanjay Saraf and Ravi S. Parihar, "Sushruta: The First Plastic Surgeon in 600 B.C.," *Internet Journal of Plastic Surgery*, 2007, vol 4, no 2. http://www.ispub.com/journal/the_internet_journal_of_plastic_surgery/volume_4_number_2_40/article/sushruta_the_first_plastic_surgeon_in_600_b_c.html. Accessed September 27, 2008.

43 "Suture materials were made": P. S. Chari, "Sushruta and Our Heritage," *Indian Journal of Plastic Surgery*, 2003, vol 36, no 1, 4–13. http://www.ijps.org/article.asp?issn=0970-0358;year=2003;volume=36;issue=1;spage=4;epage=13;aulast=chari. Accessed July 7, 2007.

43 "When these Sanskrit writings": Kaviraj Kunja Lal Bhishagratna, *An English Translation of the Sushruta Samhita*, Calcutta, 1907. http://www.archive.org/details/englishtranslati00susruoft. Accessed September 27, 2008.

43 "The archives of Boston's": N. M. Greene, "Anesthesia and the Development of Surgery, 1846–1896," *Anesth. Analg.*, 1979, vol 58, 5. Cited in John T. Sullivan, American Society of Anesthesiologists Newsletter, September 1996, 1. http://www.asahq.org/Newsletters/1996/09_96/Feature2.htm. Accessed January 21, 2007.

44 "The physician recalled": J. J. Pullen, *The Men Who Brought Us Anesthesia*, 1976. Available in Massachusetts General Hospital Archives, Boston, Massachusetts. Cited in John T. Sullivan, American Society of Anesthesiologists Newsletter, September 1996, 1. http://www.asahq.org/Newsletters/1996/09_96/Feature2.htm. Accessed January 21, 2007.

44 "When the patient awakened": Massachusetts General Hospital, http://neurosurgery.mgh.harvard.edu/History/gift/htm. Accessed May 26, 2008.

44 "The *People's Journal* of London": Massachusetts General Hospital, http://neurosurgery.mgh.harvard.edu/History/gift.htm. Accessed May 26, 2008.

44 "His accounts of surgical practice": Stephen Smith, "The Comparative Results of Operations in Bellevue Hospital," in George Shrady, ed., *Medical Record*, New York: William Wood and Co., 1885, 427–428.

45 "Yet the surgeon reported": Joseph Lister, "Antiseptic Principle of the Practice of Surgery," 1867, http://www.fordham.edu/
halsall/mod/1867lister.html. Accessed May 26, 2008.

46 "He defines unnecessary surgery this way": Lucian Leape, "Unnecessary Surgery," *Annual Review of Public Health*, vol. 13, May
1992, 366.

47 "Dr. Leape reviewed published research": Leape, "Unnecessary
Surgery," 374.

47 "Where rigorous scientific evidence": Lucian Leape, "Unnecessary Surgery," *Health Services Research,"* vol 3, August 1989,
351.

47 "As many as one-third of people": Lucian L. Leape, et al., "Effect
of Variability in the Interpretation of Coronary Angiograms on
the Appropriateness of Use of Coronary Revascularization Procedures," *American Heart Journal*, vol 139, no 1, part 1, January
2000, 111.

47 "In addition, 17 percent": Leape, et al., "Effect of Variability,"
112.

48 "The number of people on Medicare": James Weinstein, et al.,
"United States' Trends and Regional Variations in Lumbar Spine
Surgery: 1992–2003," *Spine*, vol 31, no 23, 2006, 2707–2714.

48 "Yet the operation is": Ivar Brox, et al., "Randomized Clinical
Trial of Lumbar Instrumented Fusion and Cognitive Intervention
and Exercises in Patients with Chronic Low Back Pain and Disc
Degeneration," *Spine*, vol 28, 2003, 1913–1921.

48 "When injured workers in Washington State": Sham Maghout
Juratli et al., "Lumbar Fusion Outcomes in Washington State
Workers' Compensation," *Spine*, vol 31, no 23, 2006, 2715.

49 "Yet the surgeons who perform these operations": Bill Steiger,
"Doctors Say Many Obstacles Block Paths to Patient Safety," *Physician Executive*, May–June 2007, 10.

50 "They found that children with persistent ear infections": Jack L.
Paradise, et al., "Tympanostomy Tubes and Developmental Outcomes at 9 to 11 Years of Age," *New England Journal of Medicine*,
vol 356, no 3, January 18, 2007, 248.

50 "They concluded that": Salomeh Keyhani, et al., "Overuse of Tympanostomy Tubes in New York Metropolitan Area: Evidence from
Five Hospital Cohort," *British Medical Journal*, vol. 337, 2008,
1607. Also see Salomeh Keyhani, et al., "Clinical Characteristics
of New York City Children Who Received Tympanostomy Tubes
in 2002," *Pediatrics*, vol 121, no 1, 24–33.

50 "Thousands of women may die prematurely": William H. Parker,
et al., "Ovarian Conservation at the Time of Hysterectomy for Be-

nign Disease," *Obstetrics and Gynecology*, August 2005, vol 106, no 2, 219–226.

51 "The predominant teaching": David Olive, "Dogma, Skepsis, and the Analytic Method: The Role of Prophylactic Oophorectomy at the Time of Hysterectomy," *Obstetrics and Gynecology*, vol 106, no 2, August 2005, 106, 214.

51 "We thought we would find": William Parker, "About Our Study," http://www.ovaryresearch.com/study.htm. Accessed July 4, 2009.

52 "By the time": Parker, "About Our Study."

53 "About twenty years ago": Institute of Medicine, *Assessing Medical Technologies*, Washington, D.C., 1985, 6. The report cites the Congressional Office of Technology Assessment, which is the source of this statistic.

53 "He concluded that": David M. Eddy, "Evidence-Based Medicine: A Unified Approach," *Health Affairs*, vol 24, no 1, 2005, 9–17. http://content.healthaffairs.org/cgi/content/full/24/1/9. Accessed February 28, 2009.

53 "When different physicians are recommending": Eddy, "Evidence-Based Medicine," 9–17.

54 "Dr. James Reinertsen": James Reinertsen, "Zen and the Art of Physician Autonomy Maintenance," *Annals of Internal Medicine*, vol 138, no 12, June 17, 2003, 992–995.

54 "Dr. Owen Wangensteen and colleagues": Owen Wangensteen, "The Stomach Since the Hunters: Gastric Temperature and Peptic Ulcer," lecture delivered at the Royal College of Surgeons of England, January 10, 1962.

55 "According to *Time*": "To Freeze or Not to Freeze," *Time*, November 8, 1963, http://www.time.com/time/magazine/print-out/0,8816,897016,00.html. Accessed January 4, 2007.

55 "The *New York Times* reported": Robert Plumb, "Freezing Method in Ulcers Queried: Surgeons Voice Reservation on Widely Used System," *New York Times*, October 29, 1963, 38.

58 "In 1988 researchers at the Rand Corporation": C. M. Winslow, D. H. Solomon, M. R. Chassin, J. Kosecoff, N. J. Merrick, and R. H. Brook, "The Appropriateness of Carotid Endarterectomy," *New England Journal of Medicine*, vol 318, no 12, March 24, 1988, 721–727.

59 "They reviewed more than 9,500 medical records": E. A. Halm, S. Tuhrim, J. J. Wang, M. Rojas, E. L. Hannan, and M. R. Chassin, "Has Evidence Changed Practice? Appropriateness of Carotid Endarterectomy After the Clinical Trials," *Neurology*, vol 68, 2007, 187–194, http://www.neurology.org/cgi/content/abstract/68/3/187. Accessed February 10, 2007.

60 "Researchers wondered whether chest x-rays": American Cancer Society, "How Is Small-cell Lung Cancer Staged?" Cancer Reference Information, 6. http://www.cancer.org/docroot/CRI/content/CRI_2_4_3x_How_Is_Small_Cell_Lung_Cancer_Staged.asp. Accessed October 4, 2008.

60 "In the 1970s, randomized clinical trials": Institute of Medicine, *Fulfilling the Potential of Cancer Prevention and Early Detection*, Washington, D.C., National Academy of Sciences, 2003, 292. http://orsted.nap.edu/openbook/0309082544/gifmid/292.gif. Accessed February 18, 2007.

60 "In the studies conducted at the Mayo Clinic": Institute of Medicine, *Fulfilling the Potential*, 274.

61 "Based on this research": Institute of Medicine, *Fulfilling the Potential*, 274.

61 "Dr. Reinertsen encourages legislators": Reinertsen, "Zen," 992–995.

4: The Human Face of "Too Much"

65 "Looking back on his painful ordeal": Donald Berwick, "My Right Knee," Plenary address at the IHI 15th Annual National Forum on Quality Improvement in Health Care, December 4, 2003, 17–18.

69 "The rate of heart bypass surgery in his community": *Dartmouth Atlas of Health Care*: Studies of Surgical Variation, Cardiac Surgery Report, 13, 14. http://www.dartmouthatlas.org/atlases/Cardiac_report_2005.pdf. Accessed June 21, 2008.

70 "They do not, and in fact": *Dartmouth Atlas*, Cardiac Surgery Report, 13–14.

77 "During the office visit she remembers": See Mary Anne Wyatt, "Mary Anne," in Lise Cloutier-Steele, ed., *Misinformed Consent: Women's Stories About Unnecessary Hysterectomy*, 2003, Chester, N.J.: Old Decade, 2003, 181–190.

80 "She says she lives in a body": Wyatt in Cloutier-Steele, *Misinformed Consent*, 187.

82 "And what of that *other*, the patient": Richard Selzer, *Mortal Lessons: Notes on the Art of Surgery*, New York: Harcourt, 1976, 101–102.

5: Are You Being Nuked?

85 "Dr. Thomas Graboys of Harvard Medical School calculated the impact": Thomas B. Graboys, "The Economics of Screening Joggers," *New England Journal of Medicine*, vol 301, no 19, November 8, 1979, 1067.

86 "In 2005 the National Institutes of Health (NIH) included x-rays": Report on Carcinogens, 11th ed., National Toxicology Program,

National Institutes of Health, January 31, 2005. http://ntp.niehs .nih.gov/files/11thROC_factsheet_1-31-05.pdf. Accessed May 31, 2009.

87 "One-third of adults who have the tests": David J. Brenner and Eric J. Hall, "Computed Tomography—An Increasing Source of Radiation Exposure," *New England Journal of Medicine,* vol 357, no 22, November 29, 2007, 2277–2284. http://content.nejm.org/ cgi/content/full/357/22/2277. Accessed May 26, 2008.

87 "Among children, more than one million have": Brenner and Hall, "Computed Tomography." See also Panel Discussion, *Pediatric Radiology*, vol 32, 2002, 242–244. Published online March 6, 2002. http://www.springerlink/com/content/p1wwgcyddu2wqrjy/ fulltext.pdf. Accessed October 4, 2008.

88 "He found that the radiation dose": David J. Brenner, August 31, 2004, press release of the Radiological Society of North America.

88 "Among 45-year-olds": David J. Brenner and Carl D. Elliston, "Estimated Radiation Risks Potentially Associated with Full-Body CT Screening," *Radiology*, vol 232, September 2004, 738.

90 "Closer to home, Mettler has studied": Fred A. Mettler, et al., "Effective Doses in Radiology and Diagnostic Nuclear Medicine: A Catalog," *Radiology,* vol 248, 2008, 254. http://radiology.rsnajnls. org/cgi/content/abstract/248/1/254. Accessed April 11, 2009.

90 "In fact the American College of Radiology concludes": E. Stephen Amis, et al., "American College of Radiology White Paper on Radiation Dose in Medicine," *Journal of the American College of Radiology*, vol 4, 2007, 272.

6: Uncertainty

98 "According to historical accounts": This history is reported by Tobias Lear, Journal Account of George Washington's Last Illness and Death. http://gwpapers.virginia.edu/project/exhibit/mourning/lear.html. Accessed May 31, 2008.

99 "Throughout the day Washington's health deteriorated": James Craik and Elisha Dick, Account of Washington's Last Illness and Death, December 21, 1799, in Papers of George Washington, University of Virginia. http://gwpapers.virginia.edu/project/exhibit/ mourning/craik.html. Accessed November 18, 2006.

99 "Washington understood this to be true": Lear, Washington's Last Illness and Death.

100 "About ten o'clock Saturday night": Lear, Washington's Last Illness and Death.

100 "Today we know that many of their methods were wrong": White McKenzie Wallenborn, "George Washington's Terminal Illness,"

March 29, 1999, 2. http://gwpapers.virginia.edu/articles/wallen born.html, accessed May 31, 2008.

100 "He had sued the editor": D. M. Morens, "Death of a President," *New England Journal of Medicine*, vol. 341, no 24, December 9, 1999, 1845–1850.

101 "I saw no inconvenience": Benjamin Rush, "Account of the Bilious Remitting Yellow Fever as It Appeared in the City of Philadelphia in the Year 1793." Philadelphia: Thomas Dobson, 1794, 271–272. http://deila.dickinson.edu/cdm4/document .php?cisoroot=/ownwords&cisoptr=20237. Accessed August 29, 2009.

101 "Cobbett described Rush's practice": See Lisbeth Haakonssen, *Medicine and Morals in the Enlightenment*, Amsterdam: Rodopi, 1997, 199.

101 "On the 14th of December": Cited in N. E. Davies, G. H. Davies, and E. D. Sanders, "William Cobbett, Benjamin Rush, and the Death of General Washington," *Journal of the American Medical Association*, vol 249, no 7, February 18, 1983, 914.

102 "With the benefit of hindsight": White McKenzie Wallenborn, "George Washington's Terminal Illness," March 29, 1999, http:// gwpapers.virginia.edu/articles/wallenborn.html, accessed May 31, 2008.

102 "I proposed to attempt his restoration": Papers of William Thornton, ed. by C. M. Harris, Charlottesville: University Press of Virginia, 1995, vol 1, 528. Also at http://gwpapers.virginia.edu/ project/exhibit/mourning/thornton.html. Accessed November 18, 2006.

104 "Abraham Lincoln once said": Abraham Lincoln, State of the Union Address, December 1, 1862. http://www.infoplease.com/t/ hist/state-of-the-union/74.html. Accessed July 2, 2008.

104 "When physicians and other": Mark R. Chassin, "Is Health Care Ready for Six Sigma Quality?" *Milbank Quarterly*, vol 76, no 4, 1998. http://www.milbank.org/quarterly/764featchas.html. Accessed July 8, 2007.

107 "He found that one of four": Brendan Reilly, "Physical Examination in the Care of Medical Inpatients: An Observational Study," *Lancet*, vol 362, October 4, 2003, 1100.

108 "The human gathering of intelligence": Brendan Reilly, Christopher Smith, and Brian Lucas, "Physical Examination: Bewitched, Bothered, and Bewildered," *Medical Journal of Australia*, vol 182, no 8, April 18, 2005, 376.

109 "Afterward the percentage of women": Thomas J. Smith, et al., "The Rural Cancer Oncology Program: Clinical and Financial

Analysis of Palliative and Curative Care for an Underserved Population," *Cancer Treatment Reviews*, vol 22, Supplement, 1996, 2.

109 "Selzer writes of the manner of diagnosis": Selzer, *Mortal Lessons*, 34.

110 "Between the chambers of her heart": Selzer, *Mortal Lessons*, 35.

110 "Here, then, is the doctor": Selzer, *Mortal Lessons*, 36.

7: Madison Avenue Marketing vs. Medicine: A Family's Story

113 "Of the forty-two children who had had the operation": Donald Nuss, Robert Kelly, Daniel Croitoru, and Michael Katz, "A 10-Year Review of a Minimally Invasive Technique for the Correction of Pectus Excavatum," *Journal of Pediatric Surgery*, vol 33, no 4, April 1998, 545.

115 "More than a year and a half": John Monk, "How a Hospital Failed a Boy Who Didn't Have to Die," *The State*, June 16, 2002, A1, A8–9. http://www.lewisblackman.net. Accessed May 30, 2008.

116 "The incidence of complications": Andre Hebra, Barbara Swoveland, Michael Egbert, Edward Tagge, Keith Georgeson, H. Biermann Othersen, and Donald Nuss, "Outcome Analysis of Minimally Invasive Repair of Pectus Excavatum: Review of 251 Cases," *Journal of Pediatric Surgery*, vol 35, no 2, February 2000, 256.

117 "Although previous reports suggest few complications": Scott Engum, Fred Rescorla, Karen West, Thomas Rouse, L. R. Scherer, and Jay Grosfeld, "Is the Grass Greener? Early Results of the Nuss Procedure," *Journal of Pediatric Surgery*, vol 35, no 2, February 2000, 251.

117 "Pediatric surgeons from Stanford": R. Lawrence Moss, Craig Albanese, and Marleta Reynolds, "Major Complications After Minimally Invasive Repair of Pectus Excavatum: Case Reports," *Journal of Pediatric Surgery*, vol 36, no 1, January 2001, 155.

117 "The authors concluded that the procedure": Kim Molik, Scott Engum, Frederick Rescorla, Karen West, L. R. Scherer, and Jay Grosfeld, "Pectus Excavatum Repair: Experience with Standard and Minimal Invasive Techniques," *Journal of Pediatric Surgery*, vol 36, no 2, February 2001, 324.

118 "There were no deaths": Eric Fonkalsrud, Steven Beanes, Andre Hebra, William Adamson, and Edward Tagge, "Comparison of Minimally Invasive and Modified Ravitch Pectus Excavatum Repair," *Journal of Pediatric Surgery*, vol 37, no 3 March 2002, 413.

118 "In a letter to the journal editor": letter from Helen Haskell to the editor, *Journal of Pediatric Surgery*," May 13, 2002.

119 "But the journal article did confirm": Fonkalsrud, et al., "Comparison of Minimally Invasive," 413.

119 "The article mentioned the results of the 1998 study": Avery Comarow, "Tiny Holes, Big Surgery," *U.S. News and World Report*, July 22, 2002, 56.

121 "A small but growing body": James N. Weinstein, "The Missing Piece: Embracing Shared Decision Making to Reform Health Care," *Spine*, vol 25, no 1, 2000, 1.

8: Marinated Minds

124 "Is it any wonder that": Richard A. Deyo and Donald L. Patrick, *Hope or Hype: The Obsession with Medical Advances and the High Cost of False Promises*, New York: AMACOM, 2005, 14.

125 "Schwitzer says, 'This is an amazing admission'": Gary Schwitzer, "My Report on the State of Health Journalism," March 12, 2009. http://www.healthnewsreview.org/publishers_note30.php. Accessed April 17, 2009.

127 "Dr. Eric Holmboe and his associates": Eric Holmboe, David Fiellin, Elizabeth Cusanelli, Michael Remetz, and Harlan Krumholz, "Perceptions of Benefit and Risk of Patients Undergoing First-time Elective Percutaneous Coronary Revascularization," *Journal of General Internal Medicine*, vol 15, no 9, September 2000, 634. http://www.pubmedcentral.nih.gov/articlerender.fcgi?artid=1495592. Accessed August 19, 2006.

127 "Dr. Holmboe says": Holmboe, et al., "Elective Percutaneous Coronary Revascularizations," 635.

127 "In another study": Mick Couper, presentation at Foundation for Informed Medical Decision Making meeting, February 4, 2009, Washington, D.C.

130 "The ambulance pulls up in front of the hospital": *Grey's Anatomy*, "Where the Wild Things Are," first aired Thursday, April 24, 2008.

9: The Chapter You Won't Want to Read

133 "People observed moments of silence": Richard Carter, *Breakthrough: The Saga of Jonas Salk*, New York, Trident Press, 1965, 1.

133 "We are like a donut shop": Bill Steiger, "Doctors Say Many Obstacles Block Paths to Patient Safety," Special Report: Quality of Care Survey, *Physician Executive*, May–June 2007, 6.

142 "An exception occurred when": See Alabama Medical Licensure Commission, http://www.albme.org/Documents/PublicDocs/MLC _FILES/MD.00020819.pdf. Accessed March 16, 2009.

10: Bypassing the Bypass

166 "In an interview with Diane Rehm": Interview with Art Buchwald on the *Diane Rehm Show*, February 24, 2006. http://wamu. org/programs/dr/06/02/24.php. Accessed May 31, 2008.

11: Do It with Me, Not to Me

168 "The American Cancer Society recommends": American Cancer Society Guidelines for the Early Detection of Cancer, http://www .cancer.org/docroot/ped/content/ped_2_3x_acs_cancer_detec tion_guidelines_36.asp. Accessed June 12, 2008.

168 "Older men who are likely to live": Louise C. Walter, Daniel Bertenthal, Karla Lindquist, and Badrinath R. Konety, "PSA Screening Among Elderly Men with Limited Life Expectancies," *Journal of the American Medical Association*, vol 296, no 19, November 15, 2006, 2336. http://jama.ama-assn.org/cgi/content/ full/296/19/2336. Accessed June 12, 2008.

169 "For these reasons, the authors recommended": Walter, et al., 1.

174 "No apparent differences in quality of life": Matthew W. Morgan, Raisa B. Deber, Hilary A. Llewellyn-Thomas, Peter Gladstone, R. J. Cusimano, Keith O'rourke, George Tomlinson, and Allan S. Detsky, "Randomized, Controlled Trial of an Interactive Videodisc Decision Aid for Patients with Ischemic Heart Disease," *Journal of the Society of General Internal Medicine*, vol 15, no 10, 2000, 685–693. http://www.pubmedcentral.nih.gov/articlerender. fcgi?artid=1495608. Accessed May 31, 2009.

177 "A primary care doctor in Chicago": Thomas Bodenheimer, Robert Berenson, and Paul Rudolf, "The Primary Care Specialty Income Gap: Why It Matters," *Annals of Internal Medicine*, vol 146, 2007, 301. http://www.annals.org/cgi/reprint/146/4/301.pdf. Accessed April 18, 2009.

12: Cull the Overuse, Not the People

185 "In his essay": Garrett Hardin, "The Tragedy of the Commons," *Science*, December 13, 1968. http://www.sciencemag.org/sciext/ sotp/commons.dtl. Accessed February 4, 2009.

187 "His story was reported in": Andrew Browne, "Health Crisis: Chinese Doctors Tell Patients to Pay Upfront, or No Treatment," *Wall Street Journal*, December 5, 2005, A1.

194 "According to this purported breakthrough idea": Charles R. Morris, "Why U.S. Health Care Costs Aren't Too High," *Harvard Business Review, Breakthrough Ideas for 2007*, February 2007, 50.

13: The Other Inconvenient Truth

198 "As Dr. Donald Berwick has written": Donald Berwick, foreword, in Eugene Nelson, Paul Batalden, and Marjorie Godfrey, *Quality by Design*, San Francisco: Jossey-Bass, 2007, xx.

201 "Garrett Hardin writes, 'An implicit'": Hardin, "Tragedy of the Commons."

15: Twenty Smart Ways to Protect Yourself

215 "there is no mother in the system": attributed to Helen Darling, president of the National Business Group on Health.

215 "The foundation creates": For more information, see the Foundation for Informed Medical Decision Making website, http://www.informedmedicaldecisions.org/patient_decision_aids.html. Accessed March 15, 2009.

216 "Go to the website": Go to www.dartmouthatlas.org. On the left-hand side of the home page, click on download. Scroll down to "surgical discharge rates" and under "hospital referral region" or HRR, click on 2005. The table shows large differences in the rates of back surgeries, angioplasty, heart bypass surgery, knee replacement surgery, and other procedures in more than three hundred communities in the United States.

Index

A NOTE ON THE AUTHORS

Rosemary Gibson is a writer and thought leader in American health care. At the Robert Wood Johnson Foundation for sixteen years she led a national strategy to bring palliative care into mainstream health care. She is nationally recognized for her work to advance patient safety. Ms. Gibson has also been vice president of the Economic and Social Research Institute and served as senior research associate at the American Enterprise Institute. She has been a consultant to the Medical College of Virginia and the Virginia State Legislature's Commission on Health Care. She is principal author of *Wall of Silence*, a book of narratives about medical mistakes; her articles have appeared in the *Wall Street Journal* and the *Journal of the Royal Society of Medicine*.

Janardan Prasad Singh is an economist at the World Bank and has written extensively on health care, social policy, and economic development. He has been a member of the International Advisory Council for several prime ministers of India, and has worked on economic policy at the American Enterprise Institute and on foreign policy at the United Nations. He was a member of the Board of Contributors of the *Wall Street Journal* and is co-author of *Wall of Silence*.